# Illustrated Tutorials in Clinical Ophthalmology

*Acquisitions editor:* Melanie Tait
*Development editor:* Zoë Youd
*Production controller:* Chris Jarvis
*Desk editor:* Jane Campbell
*Cover designer:* Alan Studholme

# Illustrated Tutorials in Clinical Ophthalmology

**Jack J Kanski** MD, MS, FRCS, FRCOphth

*Consultant Ophthalmic Surgeon,*
*Prince Charles Eye Unit,*
*King Edward VII Hospital,*
*Windsor*


**Anne Bolton** BIPP, DATEC

*Photography Department,*
*Prince Charles Eye Unit,*
*King Edward VII Hospital,*
*Windsor*

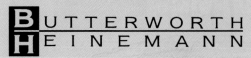

OXFORD   AUCKLAND   BOSTON   JOHANNESBURG   MELBOURNE   NEW DELHI

Butterworth-Heinemann
Linacre House, Jordan Hill, Oxford OX2 8DP
225 Wildwood Avenue, Woburn, MA 01801-2401
A division of Reed Educational and Professional Publishing Ltd

℞ A member of the Reed Elsevier plc group

First published 2001

**British Library Cataloguing in Publication Data**
Kanski, Jack J.
    Illustrated tutorials in clinical ophthalmology
    1.  Ophthalmology
    I.   Title II. Bolton, Anne III. Illustrated tutorials in clinical ophthalmology
    617.7

**Library of Congress Cataloguing in Publication Data**
A catalogue record for this book is available from the Library of Congress

ISBN 0 7506 5272 1

Printed and bound in India by Ajanta Offset

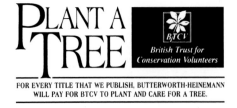

# Contents

Please note that the whole of this book appears as a Microsoft® Powerpoint® presentation on the CD-ROM enclosed with this book. Tutorials identified with 💿 on this contents list are on the CD-ROM only, they do not appear in the book.

# Preface

This book and CD-ROM are based on a series of lectures given to ophthalmologists in training at the Prince Charles Eye Unit. They contain a summary of important facts which can be used both as a guide for revision purposes as well as a framework for acquiring more in-depth knowledge of ophthalmology.

The CD-ROM contains more information than the book. The more important topics are included in the book and these are complemented by additional information which appears on the CD-ROM only.

Jack J Kanski
Anne Bolton
Windsor

# Abbreviations

| | | | | |
|---|---|---|---|---|
| AC/A | accommodative convergence to accommodation (ratio) | | ICG | indocyanine green |
| AC-IOL | anterior chamber intraocular lens | | IDD | insulin-dependent diabetes |
| AIDS | acquired immune deficiency syndrome | | IOID | idiopathic orbital inflammatory disease |
| ALT | argon laser trabeculoplasty | | IOL | intraocular lens |
| AMD | age-related macular degeneration | | IOP | intraocular pressure |
| ANA | antinuclear antibodies | | JIC | juvenile idiopathic arthritis |
| APD | afferent pupillary defect | | | |
| ARC | abnormal retinal correspondence | | KP | keratic precipitates |
| A-V | arteriovenous | | | |
| | | | M | male |
| BCC | basal cell carcinoma | | MRI | magnetic resonance imaging |
| BSV | binocular single vision | | | |
| | | | NVD | neovascularization of disc |
| CF | counting fingers | | NVE | neovascularization elsewhere |
| CMO | cystoid macular oedema | | | |
| CMV | cytomegalovirus | | PAM | primary acquired melanosis |
| CNS | central nervous system | | PAN | polyarteritis nodosa |
| CNV | choroidal neovascularization | | PAS | peripheral anterior synechiae |
| CRVO | central retinal vein occlusion | | PC-IOL | posterior chamber intraocular lens |
| CSF | cerebrospinal fluid | | PED | pigment epithelial detachment |
| CT | computed tomography | | PHVE | persistent hyperplastic primary vitreous |
| DNA | deoxyribonucleic acid | | PL | perception of light |
| | | | POAG | primary open-angle glaucoma |
| EOG | electro-oculography | | PRP | panretinal photocoagulation |
| ERG | electroretinography | | PVD | posterior vitreous detachment |
| ESR | erythrocyte sedimentation rate | | | |
| | | | RD | retinal detachment |
| F | female | | ROP | retinopathy of maturity |
| FA | fluorescein angiography | | RP | retinitis pigmentosa |
| FAZ | foveal avascular zone | | RPE | retinal pigment epithelium |
| | | | SLE | systemic lupus erythematosus |
| HM | hand movements | | TB | tuberculosis |
| | | | VA | visual acuity |

# BENIGN EYELID LESIONS

### 1. Nodules
- Chalazion
- Acute hordeola
- Molluscum contagiosum
- Xanthelasma

### 2. Cysts
- Cyst of Moll
- Cyst of Zeis
- Hidrocystoma
- Sebaceous cyst

### 3. Tumours
- Viral wart
- Keratoses
- Keratoacanthoma
- Naevi
- Capillary haemangioma
- Port-wine stain
- Pyogenic granuloma
- Cutaneous horn

## 1. Nodules

### Chalazion

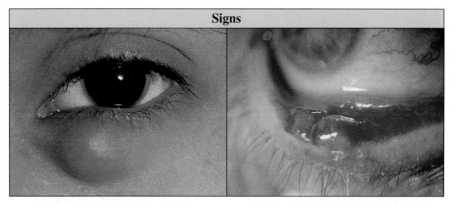

- Painless, roundish, firm lesion within tarsal plate
- May rupture through conjunctiva and cause granuloma

**Histology**

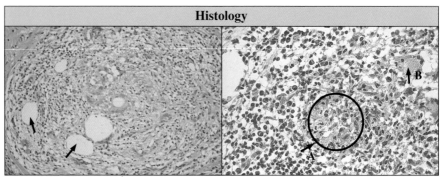

- Multiple, round spaces previously containing fat with surrounding granulomatous inflammation
- Epithelioid cells (A)
- Multinucleated giant cells (B)

**Treatment**

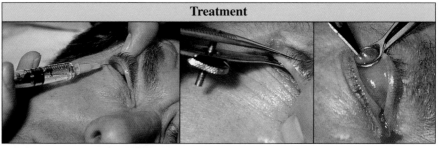

- Injection of local anaesthetic
- Insertion of clamp
- Incision and curettage

**Acute hordeola**

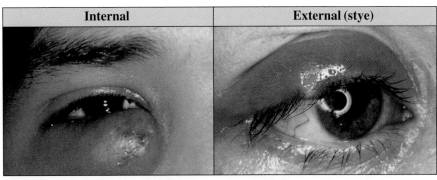

| Internal | External (stye) |
|---|---|

- *Staph.* abscess of meibomian glands
- Tender swelling within tarsal plate
- May discharge through skin or conjunctiva

- *Staph.* abscess of lash follicle and associated gland of Zeis or Moll
- Tender swelling at lid margin
- May discharge through skin

**Molluscum contagiosum**

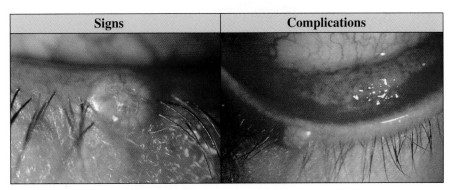

| Signs | Complications |
|---|---|

- Painless, waxy, umbilicated nodule
- May be multiple in AIDS patients

- Chronic follicular conjunctivitis
- Occasionally superficial keratitis

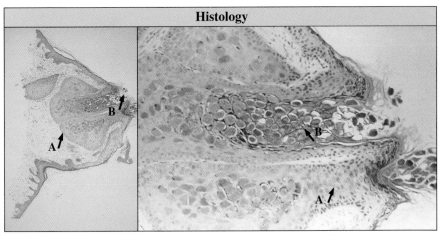

| Histology |
|---|

- Circumscribed lesion (A)
- Surface covered by normal epithelium except in centre (B)

- Lobules of hyperplastic epithelium (A)
- Intracytoplasmic (Henderson–Patterson) inclusion bodies (B)
- Deep within lesion bodies are small and eosinophilic
- Near surface bodies are larger and basophilic

**Xanthelasma**

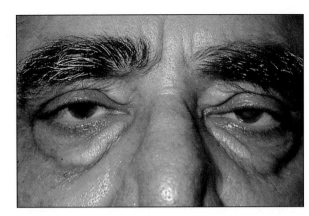

- Common in elderly or those with hypercholesterolaemia
- Yellowish, subcutaneous plaques containing cholesterol and lipid
- Usually bilateral and located medially

## 2. Cysts

**Cyst of Moll**
**Cyst of Zeis**
**Hidrocystoma**
**Sebaceous cyst**

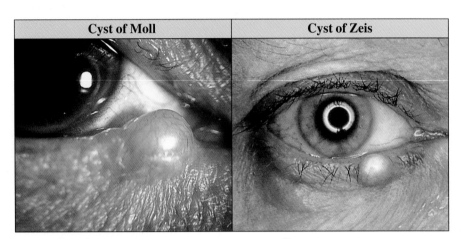

| Cyst of Moll | Cyst of Zeis |
| --- | --- |

- Translucent
- On anterior lid margin

- Opaque
- On anterior lid margin

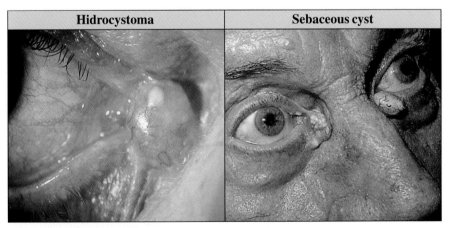

| Hidrocystoma | Sebaceous cyst |
| --- | --- |

- Similar to cyst of Moll
- Not confined to lid margin

- Cheesy contents
- Frequently at inner canthus

## 3. Tumours

**Viral wart**

| Pedunculated | Sessile |
|---|---|

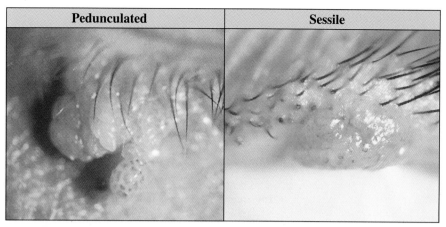

- Most common benign lid tumour
- Raspberry-like surface

| Histology |
|---|

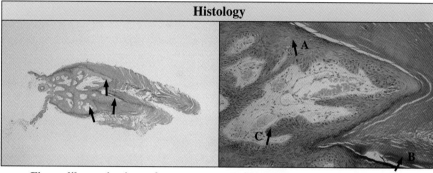

- Finger-like projections of fibrovascular connective tissue
- Epidermis shows acanthosis (A) (increased thickness) and hyperkeratosis (B)
- Rete ridges are elongated and bent inwards (C)

**Keratoses**

| Seborrhoeic | Actinic |
|---|---|

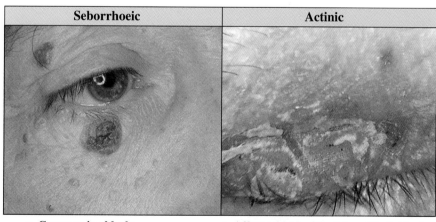

- Common in elderly
- Discrete, greasy, brown lesion
- Friable verrucous surface
- Flat 'stuck-on' appearance

- Affects elderly, fair-skinned individuals
- Most common pre-malignant skin lesion
- Rare on eyelids
- Flat, scaly, hyperkeratotic lesion

**Keratoacanthoma**

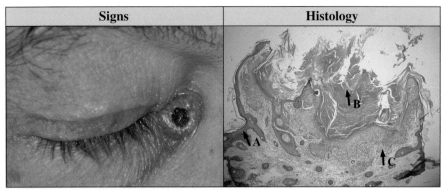

| Signs | Histology |
|---|---|

- Uncommon, fast-growing nodule
- Acquires rolled edges and keratin-filled crater
- Involutes spontaneously within 1 year

- Lesion above surface epithelium (A)
- Central keratin-filled crater (B)
- Chronic inflammatory cellular infiltration of dermis (C)

**Naevi**

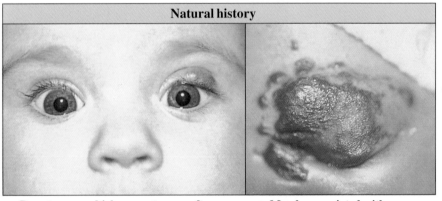

- Appearance and classification determined by location within skin
- Tend to become more pigmented at puberty

| Intradermal | Junctional | Compound |
|---|---|---|

- Elevated
- May be non-pigmented
- No malignant potential

- Flat, well-circumscribed
- Pigmented
- Low malignant potential

- Has both intradermal and junctional components

**Capillary haemangioma**

**Natural history**

- Rare tumour which presents soon after birth
- Starts as small, red lesion, most frequently on upper lid
- Blanches with pressure and swells on crying

- May be associated with intraorbital extension
- Grows quickly during first year
- Begins to involute spontaneously during second year

## Periocular haemangioma

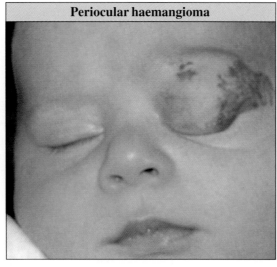

*Treatment options*
- Steroid injection in most cases
- Surgical resection in selected cases

*Occasional systemic associations*
- High-out heart failure
- Kasabach–Merritt syndrome– thrombocytopenia, anaemia and reduced coagulant factors
- Maffuci syndrome–skin haemangiomas, enchondromas and bowing of long bones

## Histology

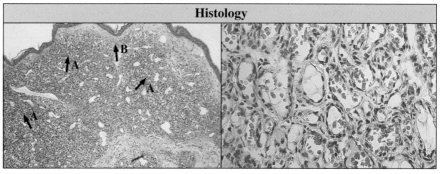

- Lobules of capillaries (A)
- Fine fibrous septae (B)

- Lobules under high magnification

**Port-wine stain**

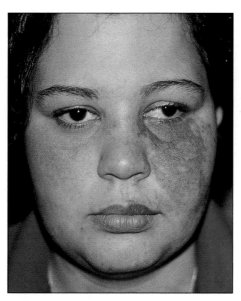

- Rare, congenital subcutaneous lesion
- Segmental and usually unilateral
- Does not blanch with pressure

*Associations*
- Ipsilateral glaucoma in 30%
- Sturge–Weber or Klippel– Trenaunay–Weber syndrome in 5%

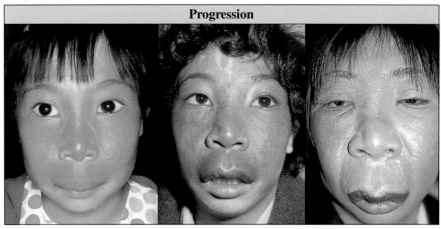

| Progression | | |
|---|---|---|
| • Initially red and flat | • Subsequent darkening and hypertrophy of skin | • Skin becomes coarse, nodular and friable |

**Pyogenic granuloma**

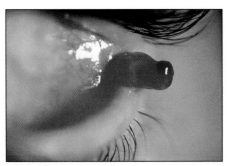

- Usually antedated by surgery or trauma
- Fast-growing pinkish, pedunculated or sessile mass
- Bleeds easily

**Cutaneous horn**

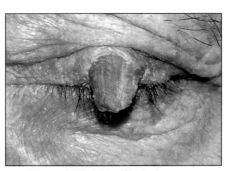

- Uncommon, horn-like lesion protruding through skin
- May be associated with underlying actinic keratosis or squamous cell carcinoma

# MALIGNANT EYELID TUMOURS

1. **Basal cell carcinoma**

2. **Squamous cell carcinoma**

3. **Meibomian gland carcinoma**

4. **Melanoma**

5. **Kaposi sarcoma**

6. **Merkel cell carcinoma**

7. **Treatment**

## 1. Basal cell carcinoma

**IMPORTANT FACTS**

1. Most common human malignancy
2. Usually affects the elderly
3. Slow-growing, locally invasive
4. Does not metastasize
5. 90% occur on head and neck
6. Of these, 10% involve eyelids
7. Accounts for 90% of eyelid malignancies

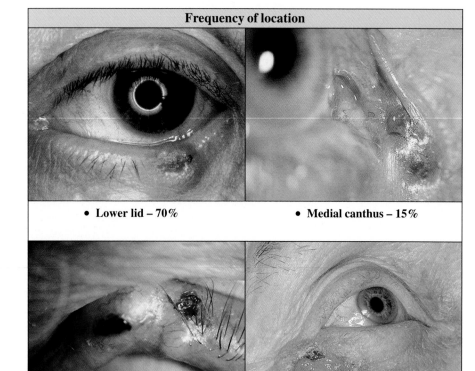

Frequency of location

- Lower lid – 70%
- Medial canthus – 15%
- Upper lid – 10%
- Lateral canthus – 5%

| Nodular | |
|---|---|
| **Early** | **Advanced** |

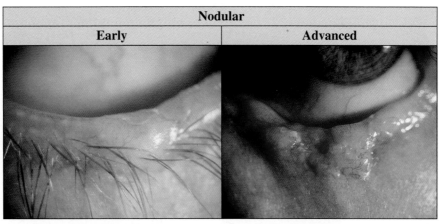

| | |
|---|---|
| • **Shiny, indurated nodule**<br>• **Surface vascularization** | • **Slow progression**<br>• **May destroy large portion of eyelid** |

| Ulcerative (rodent ulcer) | |
|---|---|
| **Early** | **Advanced** |

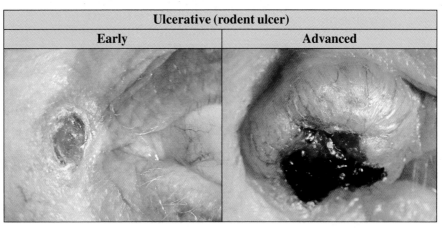

| | |
|---|---|
| • **Chronic ulceration** | • **Raised rolled edges and bleeding** |

| Sclerosing | |
|---|---|
| **Early** | **Advanced** |

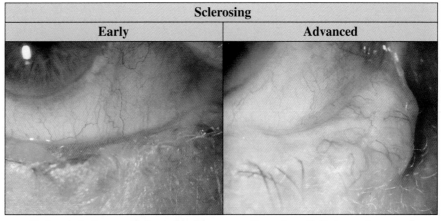

| | |
|---|---|
| • **Indurated plaque with loss of lashes**<br>• **May mimic chronic blepharitis** | • **Spreads radially beneath normal epidermis**<br>• **Margins impossible to delineate** |

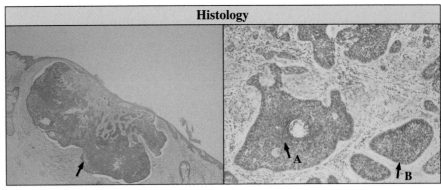

| Histology |
|---|

- Downgrowth from epidermis of small, dark atypical basal cells
- Cell nests in fibrous stoma (A)
- Peripheral palisading (B)

## 2. Squamous cell carcinoma

- ● Less common but more aggressive than BCC
- ● May arise *de novo* or from actinic keratosis
- ● Predilection for lower lid

| Nodular | Ulcerative |
|---|---|

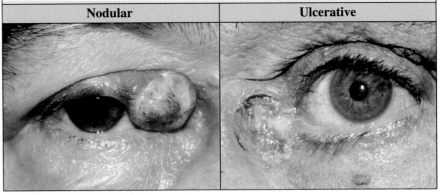

- Hard, hyperkeratotic nodule
- May develop crusting fissures
- No surface vascularization
- Red base
- Borders sharply defined, indurated and elevated

| Histology |
|---|

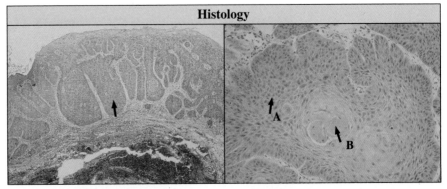

- Variable sized groups of atypical epithelial cells within dermis
- Prominent nuclei and abundant acidophilic cytoplasm (A)
- Keratin 'pearl' (B)

## 3. Meibomian gland carcinoma

- Very rare aggressive tumour with 10% mortality
- Predilection for upper lid

### Nodular

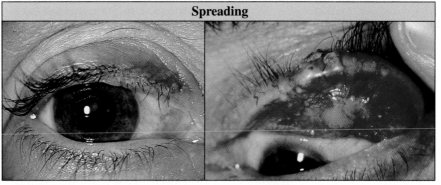

- Hard nodule; may mimic a chalazion
- Very large tumour

### Spreading

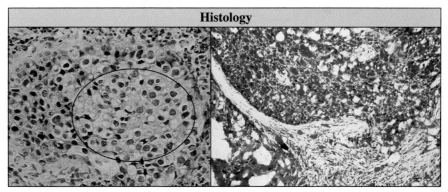

- Diffuse thickening of lid margin and loss of lashes
- Conjunctival invasion; may mimic chronic conjunctivitis

### Histology

- Cells contain foamy vacuolated cytoplasm and large hyperchromatic nuclei
- Cells stain positive for fat

## 4. Melanoma

| Nodular | Superficial spreading | From lentigo maligna (Hutchinson freckle) |
|---|---|---|

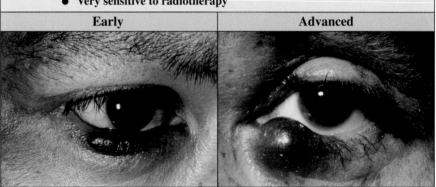

- Blue-black nodule with normal surrounding skin
- May be non-pigmented

- Plaque with irregular outline
- Variable pigmentation

- Affects elderly
- Slowly expanding pigmented macule

## 5. Kaposi sarcoma

- Vascular tumour occurring in patients with AIDS
- Usually associated with advanced disease
- Very sensitive to radiotherapy

| Early | Advanced |
|---|---|

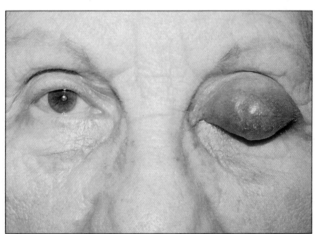

- Pink, red-violet lesion
- May ulcerate and bleed

## 6. Merkel cell carcinoma

- Highly malignant with frequent metastases at presentation
- Fast-growing, violaceous, well-demarcated nodule
- Intact overlying skin
- Predilection for upper eyelid

## 7. Treatment options

### TREATMENT OPTIONS

1. **Surgical excision**
   - Method of choice
2. **Radiotherapy**
   - Small BCC not involving medial canthus
   - Kaposi sarcoma
3. **Cryotherapy**
   - Small and superficial BCC irrespective of location
   - Adjunct to surgery in selected cases

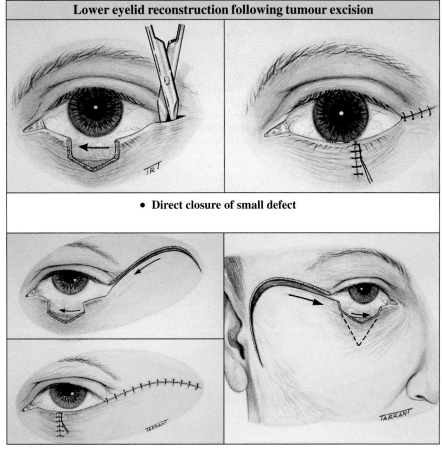

**Lower eyelid reconstruction following tumour excision**

- Direct closure of small defect

- Tenzel flap for moderate defect

- Mustarde cheek rotation flap for large defect

## Eyelid-sharing procedure

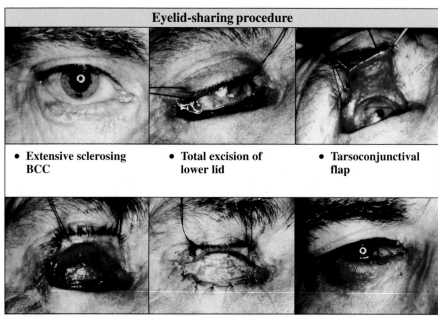

- Extensive sclerosing BCC

- Total excision of lower lid

- Tarsoconjunctival flap

- Reconstruction of posterior lamella

- Reconstruction of anterior lamella with skin graft

- Appearance after healing

# PTOSIS

## 1. Evaluation
- Pseudoptosis
- True ptosis

## 2. Classification
- Neurogenic ptosis
- Myogenic ptosis
- Aponeurotic ptosis
- Mechanical ptosis

## 3. Treatment options

## 1. Evaluation

**Pseudoptosis**

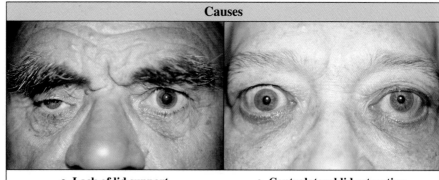

| **Causes** |
|:---:|

- Lack of lid support
- Contralateral lid retraction

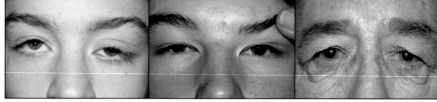

- Ipsilateral hypotropia
- Brow ptosis – excessive eyebrow skin
- Dermatochalasis – excessive eyelid skin

**True ptosis**

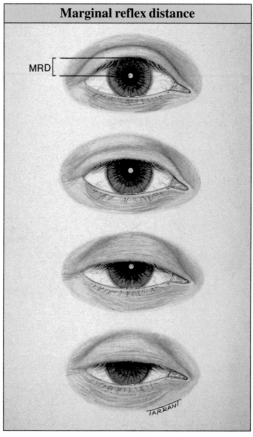

**Marginal reflex distance**

- Distance between upper lid margin and light reflex

- Mild ptosis (2 mm of droop)

- Moderate ptosis (3 mm)

- Severe ptosis (4 mm or more)

## Upper lid excursion

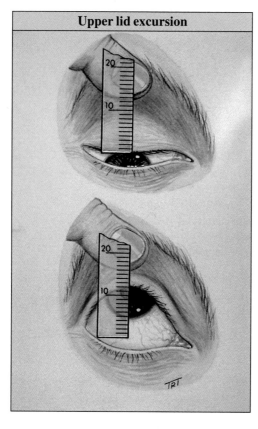

- **Reflects levator function**

- **Normal (15 mm or more)**

- **Good (12 mm or more)**

- **Fair (5–11 mm)**

- **Poor (4 mm or less)**

## Vertical fissure height

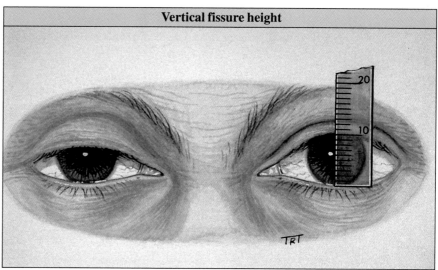

- **Distance between upper and lower lid margins**
- **Normal upper lid margin rests about 2 mm below upper limbus**
- **Normal lower lid margin rests 1 mm above lower limbus**
- **Amount of unilateral ptosis is determined by comparison**

| Upper lid crease | Pretarsal show |
|---|---|

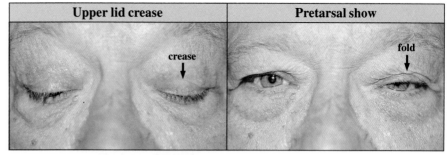

crease

fold

- Distance between lid margin and lid crease in down-gaze
- Normals – females 10 mm; males 8 mm
- Absence in congenital ptosis indicates poor levator function
- High crease suggests an aponeurotic defect

- Distance between lash line and skin fold in primary position of gaze

| Bell's phenomenon |
|---|
| ● Upward rotation of globe on lid closure |

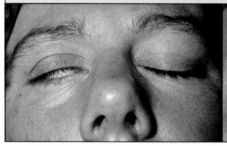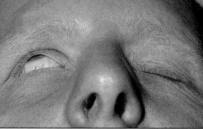

- Good

- Poor – risk of postoperative corneal exposure

2. Classification

## CLASSIFICATION

1. Neurogenic
   - Third nerve palsy
   - Third nerve misdirection
   - Horner syndrome
   - Marcus Gunn jaw-winking syndrome
2. Myogenic
   - Myasthenia gravis
   - Myotonic dystrophy
   - Ocular myopathies
   - Simple congenital
   - Blepharophimosis syndrome
3. Aponeurotic
4. Mechanical

**Neurogenic ptosis**

### Left third nerve palsy

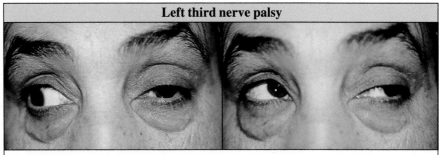

- Severe unilateral ptosis and defective adduction
- Normal abduction

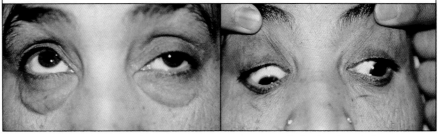

- Defective elevation
- Defective depression

- Rare, unilateral
- Aberrant regeneration following acquired third nerve palsy
- Pupil is occasionally involved
- Bizarre movements of upper lid accompany eye movements

### Right third nerve misdirection

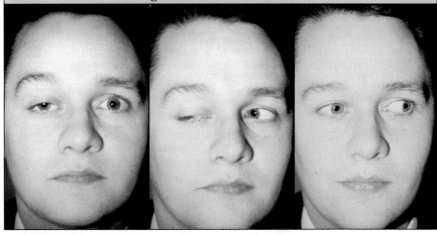

- Right ptosis in primary position
- Worse on right gaze
- Normal on left gaze

## Horner syndrome

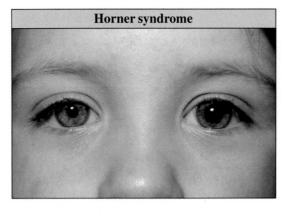

- Caused by oculosympathetic palsy
- Usually unilateral mild ptosis and miosis
- Normal pupillary reactions
- Slight elevation of lower lid
- Iris hypochromia if congenital or longstanding
- Anhydrosis if lesion is below superior cervical ganglion

## Important causes

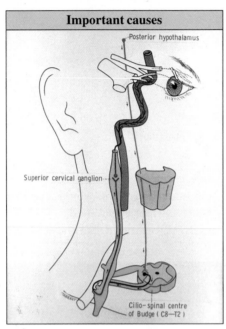

*Central*
*(first order neurone)*

- Brainstem disease (vascular, demyelination)
- Spinal cord disease (syringomyelia, tumours)

*Pre-ganglionic*
*(second order neurone)*

- Intrathoracic lesions (Pancoast tumour, aneurysm)
- Neck lesions (glands, trauma)

*Post-ganglionic*
*(third order neurone)*

- Internal carotid artery disease
- Cavernous sinus mass

## Marcus Gunn jaw-winking syndrome

- Accounts for about 5% of all cases of congenital ptosis
- Retraction or 'wink' of ptotic lid in conjunction with stimulation of ipsilateral pterygoid muscles

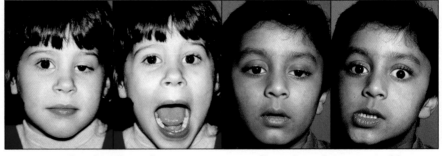

- Opening of mouth
- Contralateral movement of jaw

**Myogenic ptosis**

## MYASTHENIA GRAVIS

1. **Clinical features**
   - **Uncommon, typically affects young women**
   - **Weakness and fatiguability of voluntary musculature**
   - **Three types – ocular, bulbar and generalized**
2. **Investigations**
   - **Edrophonium test**
   - **Electromyography to confirm fatigue**
   - **Antibodies to acetylcholine receptors**
   - **CT or MRI for presence of thymoma**
3. **Treatment options**
   - **Medical – anticholinesterases, steroids and azathioprine**
   - **Thymectomy**

| Ocular myasthenia | |
|---|---|
| **Ptosis** | **Diplopia** |

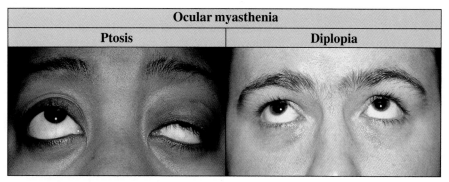

- Insidious, bilateral but asymmetrical
- Worse with fatigue and in upgaze
- Ptotic lid may show 'twitch' and 'hop' signs

- Intermittent and usually vertical

| Edrophonium test | |
|---|---|
| **Before injection** | **Positive result** |

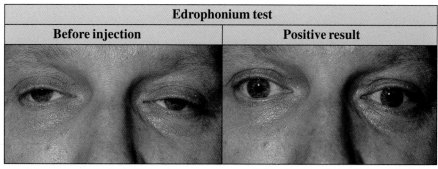

- Measure amount of ptosis or diplopia before injection
- Inject i.v. atropine 0.3 mg

- Inject i.v. test dose of edrophonium (0.2 ml – 2 mg)
- Inject remaining (0.8 ml – 8 mg) if no hypersensitivity

| Myotonic dystrophy | |
| --- | --- |
| **Release of grip difficult** | **Facial weakness and ptosis** |

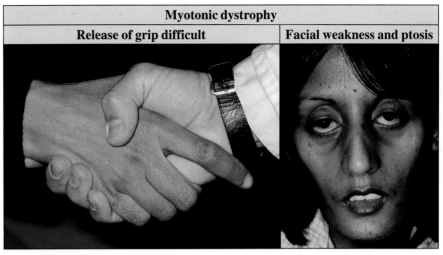

- Muscle wasting
- Involvement of tongue and pharyngeal muscles
- Ophthalmoplegia – uncommon

- Hypogonadism
- Frontal baldness in males
- Intellectual deterioration
- Presenile stellate cataracts

| Ocular myopathies | |
| --- | --- |

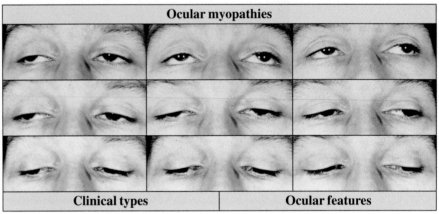

| **Clinical types** | **Ocular features** |
| --- | --- |

- Isolated
- Oculopharyngeal dystrophy
- Kearns–Sayre syndrome (pigmentary retinopathy)

- Ptosis – slowly progressive and symmetrical
- Ophthalmoplegia – slowly progressive and symmetrical (no diplopia)

## Simple congenital ptosis

- Developmental dystrophy of levator muscle
- Occasionally associated with weakness of superior rectus

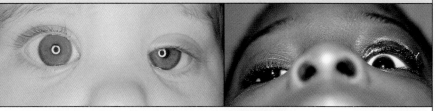

- Unilateral or bilateral ptosis of varying severity
- In downgaze ptotic eyelid is slightly higher

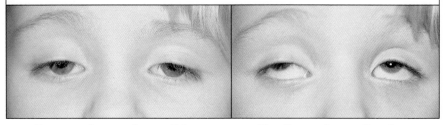

- Frequent absence of upper lid crease
- Usually poor levator function

## Blepharophimosis syndrome

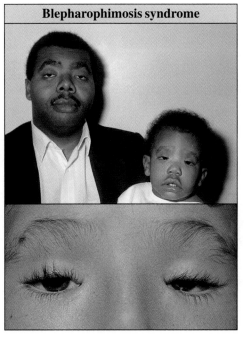

- Rare congenital disorder
- Dominant inheritance

- Moderate to severe symmetrical ptosis
- Short horizontal palpebral aperture
- Telecanthus (lateral displacement of medial canthus)
- Epicanthus inversus (lower lid fold larger than upper)
- Lateral inferior ectropion
- Poorly developed nasal bridge and hypoplasia of superior orbital rims

**Aponeurotic ptosis**

- Weakness of levator aponeurosis
- Causes – involutional, postoperative and blepharochalasis

### Mild

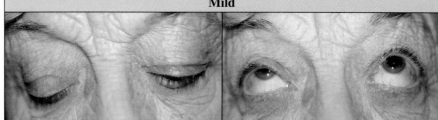

- High upper lid crease
- Good levator function

### Severe

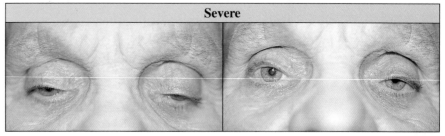

- Absent upper lid crease
- Deep sulcus

**Mechanical ptosis**

### Causes

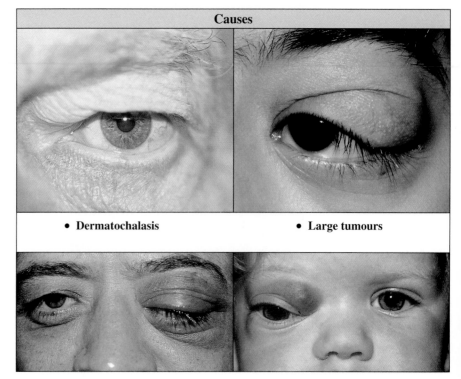

- Dermatochalasis
- Large tumours

- Severe lid oedema
- Anterior orbital lesions

## 3. Treatment options

### Fasanella–Servat procedure

● **Indicated for mild ptosis with good levator function**

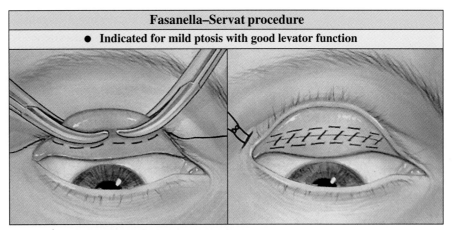

● Excision of upper border of tarsus, lower border of Müller muscle and overlying conjunctiva

### Levator resection

● **Indicated for any ptosis provided levator function is at least 5 mm**

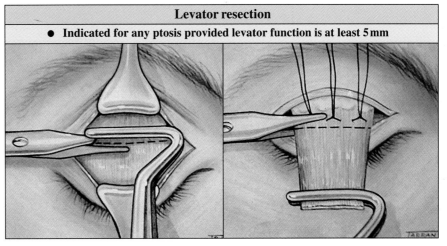

● Shortening of levator complex

● Amount determined by levator function and severity of ptosis

| Frontalis brow suspension |
| --- |
| **Main indications** |
| • Severe ptosis with poor levator function (4 mm or less)<br>• Marcus Gunn jaw-winking syndrome |

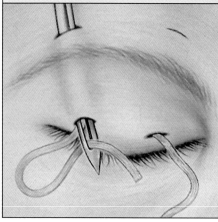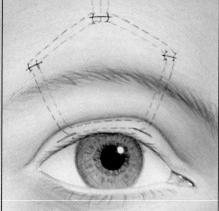

• **Attachment of tarsus to frontalis muscle with sling**

# CONJUNCTIVAL INFECTIONS

1. **Bacterial**
   - Simple bacterial conjunctivitis
   - Gonococcal keratoconjunctivitis

2. **Viral**
   - Adenoviral keratoconjunctivitis
   - Molluscum contagiosum conjunctivitis
   - Herpes simplex conjunctivitis

3. **Chlamydial**
   - Adult chlamydial keratoconjunctivitis
   - Neonatal chlamydial conjunctivitis
   - Trachoma

## 1. Bacterial

**Simple bacterial conjunctivitis**

| Signs |
|-------|

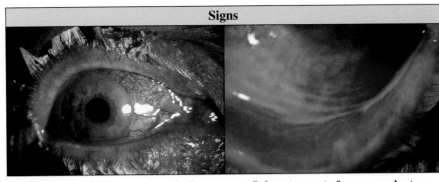

- Crusted eyelids and conjunctival injection
- Subacute onset of mucopurulent discharge

*Treatment*

- Broad-spectrum topical antibiotics

**Gonococcal keratoconjunctivitis**

| Signs | Complications |
|-------|---------------|

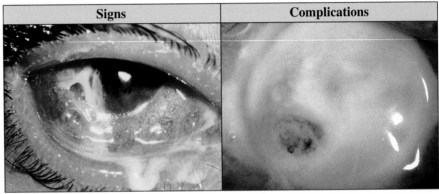

- Acute, profuse, purulent discharge, hyperaemia and chemosis
- Corneal ulceration, perforation and endophthalmitis if severe

*Treatment*

- Topical gentamicin and bacitracin
- Intravenous cefoxitin or cefotaxime

## 2. Viral

**Adenoviral keratoconjunctivitis**

| TWO TYPES |
|-----------|

1. Pharyngoconjunctival fever
   - Adenovirus types 3 and 7
   - Typically affects children
   - Upper respiratory tract infection
   - Keratitis in 30% – usually mild
2. Epidemic keratoconjunctivitis
   - Adenovirus types 8 and 19
   - Very contagious
   - No systemic symptoms
   - Keratitis in 80% of cases – may be severe

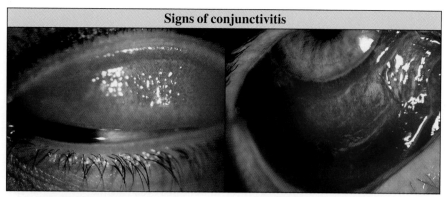

**Signs of conjunctivitis**

- Usually bilateral, acute watery discharge and follicles
- Subconjunctival haemorrhages and pseudomembranes if severe

*Treatment*
- Symptomatic

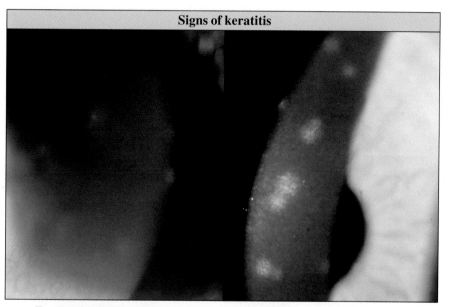

**Signs of keratitis**

- Focal, epithelial keratitis
- Transient
- Focal, subepithelial keratitis
- May persist for months

*Treatment*
- Topical steroids if visual acuity diminished by subepithelial keratitis

**Molluscum
contagiosum
conjunctivitis**

| Signs |
|---|

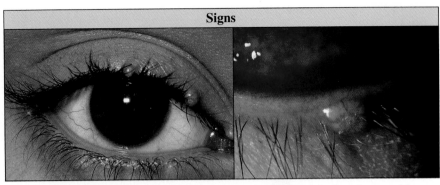

- Waxy, umbilicated eyelid nodule
- May be multiple

- Ipsilateral, chronic, mucoid discharge
- Follicular conjunctivitis

*Treatment*
- Destruction of eyelid lesion

**Herpes simplex
conjunctivitis**

| Signs |
|---|

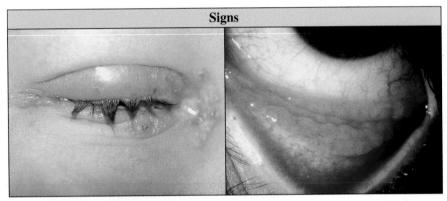

- Unilateral eyelid vesicles

- Acute follicular conjunctivitis

*Treatment*
- Topical antivirals to prevent keratitis

## 3. Chlamydial

**Adult chlamydial
keratoconjunctivitis**

- Infection with *Chlamydia trachomatis* serotypes D to K
- Concomitant genital infection is common

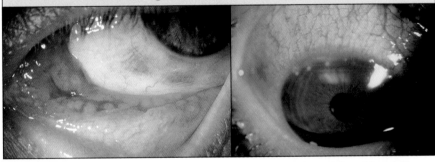

- Subacute, mucopurulent follicular conjunctivitis

- Variable peripheral keratitis

*Treatment*
- Topical tetracycline and oral tetracycline, azithromycin or erythromycin

**Neonatal chlamydial conjunctivitis**

- Presents between 5 and 19 days after birth
- May be associated with otitis, rhinitis and pneumonitis

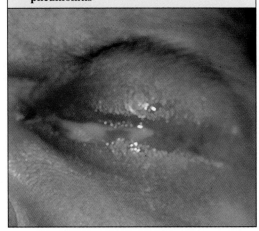

- Mucopurulent papillary conjunctivitis

*Treatment*

- Topical tetracycline and oral erythromycin

**Trachoma**

- Infection with serotypes A, B, Ba and C of *Chlamydia trachomatis*
- Fly is major vector in infection–reinfection cycle

**Progression**

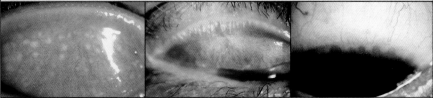

- Acute follicular conjunctivitis
- Conjunctival scarring (Arlt line)
- Herbert pits

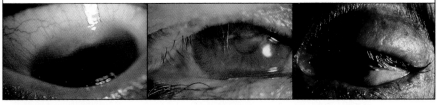

- Pannus formation
- Trichiasis
- Cicatricial entropion

*Treatment*  • Oral azithromycin

# CONJUNCTIVAL TUMOURS

## 1. Benign
- Naevus
- Papilloma
- Epibulbar dermoid
- Lipodermoid

## 2. Pre-malignant
- Intraepithelial neoplasia (carcinoma in situ)
- Primary acquired melanosis (PAM)

## 3. Malignant
- Melanoma
- Squamous cell carcinoma
- Kaposi sarcoma
- Lymphoma

## 1. Benign

**Naevus**

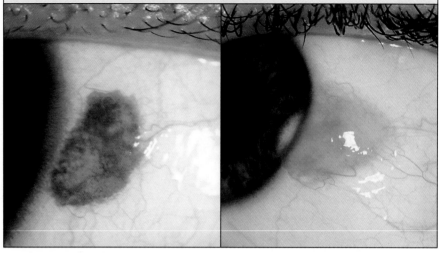

- Presents in first two decades
- Solitary, sharply demarcated
- Usually juxtalimbal

- May enlarge and become more pigmented at puberty
- 30% are almost non-pigmented

**Papilloma**

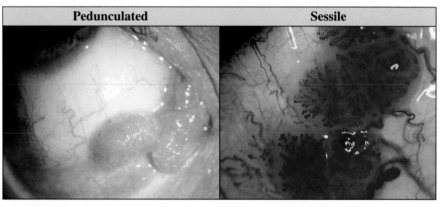

| Pedunculated | Sessile |
|---|---|

- Presents in childhood or early adulthood
- Infection with papilloma virus
- May be multiple and bilateral

- Presents in middle age
- Not caused by infection
- Single and unilateral

**Epibulbar dermoid**

| Signs | Association |
|---|---|

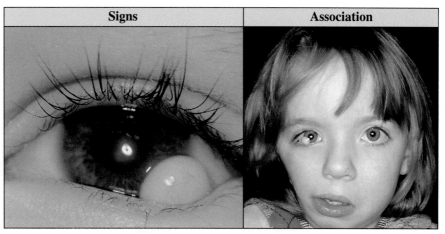

- Presents in childhood
- Smooth, soft mass
- Usually juxtalimbal

- Occasionally Goldenhar syndrome

**Lipodermoid**

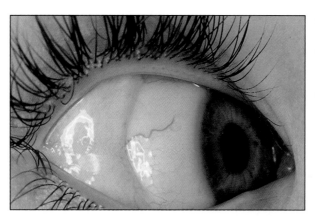

- Presents in adulthood
- Soft, movable, subconjunctival mass
- Most frequently at outer canthus

## 2. Pre-malignant

**Intraepithelial neoplasia (carcinoma in situ)**

| Signs | Progression |
|---|---|

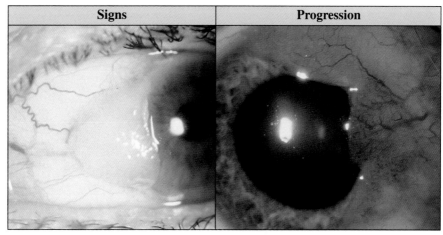

- Presents in late adulthood
- Juxtalimbal fleshy avascular mass

- May become vascular and extend onto cornea
- Malignant transformation is uncommon

**Primary acquired melanosis (PAM)**

| Signs | Types |
|---|---|
| 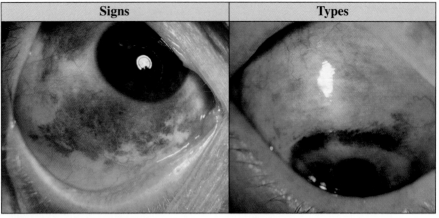 | |
| • Presents in late adulthood<br>• Unilateral, irregular areas of flat, brown pigmentation<br>• May involve any part of conjunctiva | • PAM without atypia is benign<br>• PAM with atypia is pre-malignant |

## 3. Malignant

**Melanoma**

| From PAM with atypia | From naevus | Primary |
|---|---|---|
| 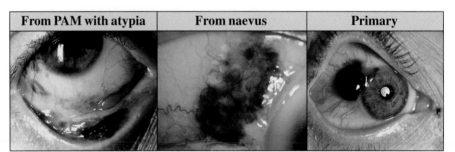 | | |
| • Most common type<br>• Sudden appearance of nodules within PAM | • Very rare<br>• Sudden increase in size or pigmentation | • Solitary nodule<br>• Frequently juxtalimbal but may be anywhere |

| Treatment of conjunctival melanoma | | |
|---|---|---|
| Localized tumour | Diffuse tumour | Orbital recurrence |
| 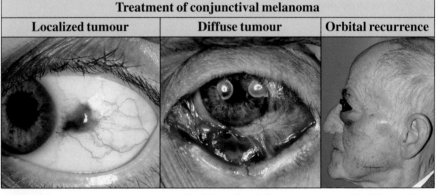 | | |
| • Excision<br>• Adjunctive cryotherapy | • Excision of nodules<br>• Adjunctive cryotherapy or mitomycin | • Excision and radiotherapy<br>• Exenteration |

**Squamous cell carcinoma**

| Signs | Progression |
|---|---|

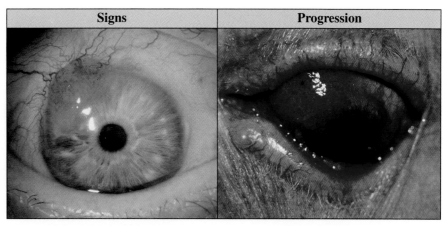

- Arises from intraepithelial neoplasia or *de novo*
- Presents in late adulthood
- Frequently juxtalimbal

- Slow-growing
- May spread extensively
- Rarely metastasizes

**Kaposi sarcoma**

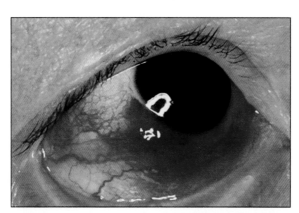

- Affects patients with AIDS
- Vascular, slow-growing tumour of low malignancy
- Very sensitive to radiotherapy
- Most frequently in inferior fornix

**Lymphoma**

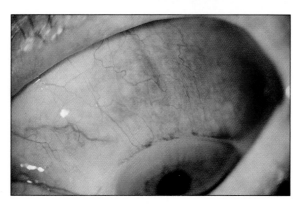

- Usually presents in adulthood
- Benign or malignant
- Salmon-coloured, subconjunctival infiltrate

# PERIPHERAL CORNEAL INFLAMMATION

1. **Marginal keratitis**

2. **Rosacea keratitis**

3. **Phlyctenulosis**

4. **Acute stromal keratitis**

**1. Marginal keratitis**

- Hypersensitivity reaction to *Staph*. exotoxins
- May be associated with *Staph*. blepharitis
- Unilateral, transient but recurrent

**Progression**

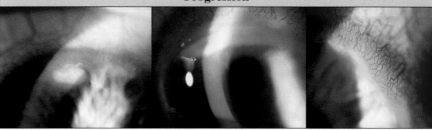

- Subepithelial infiltrate separated by clear zone
- Circumferential spread
- Bridging vascularization followed by resolution

*Treatment*
- Short course of topical steroids

**2. Rosacea keratitis**

- Affects 5% of patients with acne rosacea
- Bilateral and chronic

**Progression**

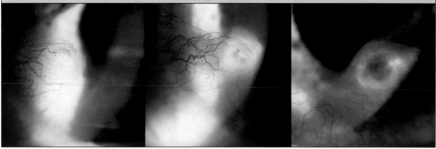

- Peripheral inferior vascularization
- Subepithelial infiltration
- Thinning and perforation if severe

*Treatment*
- Topical steroids and systemic tetracycline or doxycycline

## 3. Phlyctenu-losis

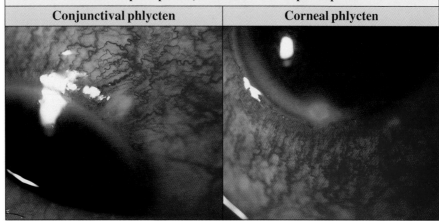

- Uncommon, unilateral – typically affects children
- Severe photophobia, lacrimation and blepharospasm

| Conjunctival phlycten | Corneal phlycten |
|---|---|

- Small pinkish-white nodule near limbus
- Usually transient and resolves spontaneously

- Starts astride limbus
- Resolves spontaneously or extends onto cornea

*Treatment*
- Topical steroids

## 4. Acute stromal keratitis

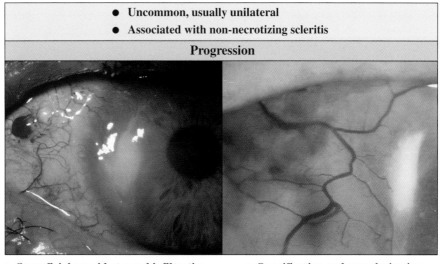

- Uncommon, usually unilateral
- Associated with non-necrotizing scleritis

| Progression |
|---|

- Superficial or mid-stromal infiltration

- Opacification and vascularization

*Treatment*
- Topical steroids and systemic non-steroidal anti-inflammatory drugs

# PERIPHERAL CORNEAL THINNING AND ULCERATION

1.  **Without systemic disease**
    - Dellen
    - Terrien marginal degeneration
    - Mooren ulcer

2.  **With systemic disease**
    - Rheumatoid arthritis
    - Wegener granulomatosis
    - Polyarteritis nodosa

## 1. Without systemic disease

**Dellen**

| Common and unilateral | |
|:---|:---|
| Innocuous | |

| Signs | Causes |
|:---:|:---:|
| | |
| • Saucer-like thinning with intact epithelium<br>• Fluorescein pooling but no staining | • Chemosis, raised limbal lesions, abnormal blinking |

*Treatment*    • Lubricants and elimination of cause

**Terrien marginal degeneration**

| Uncommon, bilateral but asymmetrical | |
|:---|:---|
| Initially asymptomatic | |

| Progression | |
|:---:|:---:|
| | |
| • Fine stromal lipid deposition separated by clear zone<br>• Mild thinning and vascularization | • Circumferential thinning and increasing astigmatism<br>• Formation of pseudo-pterygia if longstanding |

*Treatment of severe astigmatism*    • Crescent-shaped excision of gutter

**Mooren ulcer**

- Limited form – usually unilateral, affects elderly
- Progressive form – bilateral, affects younger patients

**Progression**

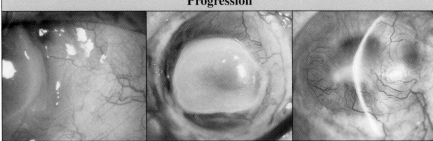

- Peripheral ulcerative keratitis
- Circumferential and central spread
- End-stage scarring and vascularization

*Treatment*
- Systemic steroids and/or cytotoxic drugs

## 2. With systemic disease

**Rheumatoid arthritis**

| Without inflammation | With inflammation |
|---|---|

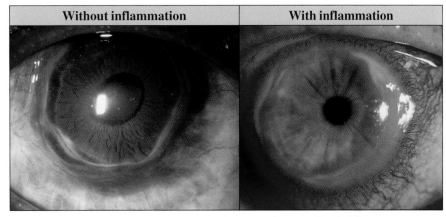

- Chronic and asymptomatic
- Circumferential thinning with intact epithelium ('contact lens cornea')

- Acute and painful
- Circumferential ulceration and infiltration

*Treatment*
- Systemic steroids and/or cytotoxic drugs

**Wegener granulomatosis**

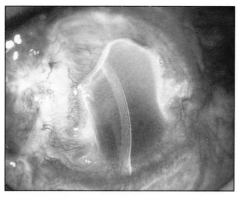

- Circumferential and central ulceration similar to Mooren ulcer

*Treatment*
- Systemic steroids and cyclophosphamide

**Polyarteritis nodosa**

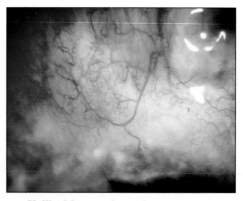

- Unlike Mooren ulcer sclera may also become involved

*Treatment*
- Systemic steroids and cyclophosphamide

# CORNEAL INFECTIONS

1. **Bacterial keratitis**

2. **Fungal keratitis**

3. **Acanthamoeba keratitis**

4. **Infectious crystalline keratitis**

5. **Herpes simplex keratitis**
   - Epithelial
   - Disciform

6. **Herpes zoster keratitis**

### 1. Bacterial keratitis

| Predisposing factors |
|---|
| • Contact lens wear |
| • Chronic ocular surface disease |
| • Corneal hypoaesthesia |
| **Progression** |

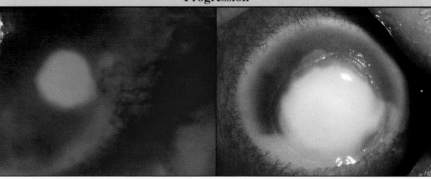

| • Expanding oval, yellow-white, dense stromal infiltrate | • Stromal suppuration and hypopyon |
|---|---|

*Treatment*  • Topical ciprofloxacin 0.3% or ofloxacin 0.3%

### 2. Fungal keratitis

| • Frequently preceded by ocular trauma with organic matter |
|---|
| **Progression** |

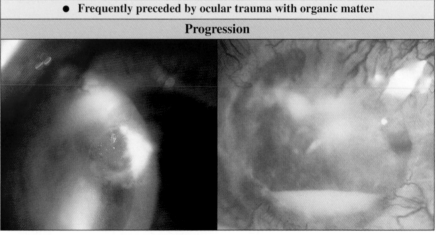

| • Greyish-white ulcer which may be surrounded by feathery infiltrates | • Slow progression and occasionally hypopyon |
|---|---|

*Treatment*  • Topical antifungal agents
  • Systemic therapy if severe
  • Penetrating keratoplasty if unresponsive

## 3. Acanthamoe-ba keratitis

- Contact lens wearers at particular risk
- Symptoms worse than signs

### Progression

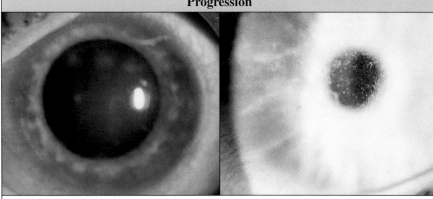

- Small, patchy anterior stromal infiltrates

- Perineural infiltrates (radial keratoneuritis)

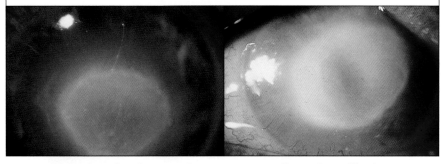

- Ulceration, ring abscess and satellite lesions

- Stromal opacification

*Treatment*
- Chlorhexidine or polyhexamethylenebiguanide

## 4. Infectious crystalline keratitis

- Very rare, indolent infection (*Strep. viridans*)
- Usually associated with long-term topical steroid use
- Particularly following penetrating keratoplasty

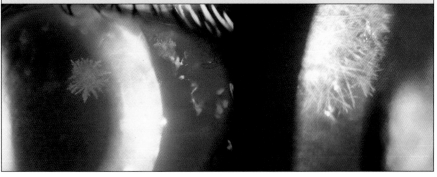

- White, branching, anterior stromal crystalline deposits

*Treatment*
- Topical antibiotics

## 5. Herpes simplex keratitis

### Epithelial

| Dendritic ulcer | Geographic ulcer |
|---|---|

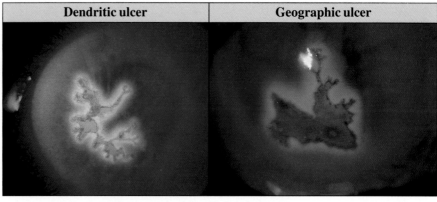

- Dendritic ulcer with terminal bulbs
- Stains with fluorescein

- May enlarge to become geographic

*Treatment*
- Aciclovir 3% ointment × 5 daily
- Trifluorothymidine 1% drops 2-hourly
- Debridement if non-compliant

### Disciform

| Signs | Association |
|---|---|

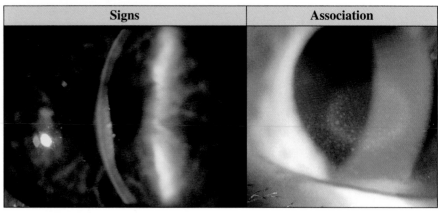

- Central epithelial and stromal oedema
- Folds in Descemet membrane
- Small keratic precipitates

- Occasionally surrounded by Wessely ring

*Treatment*
- Topical steroids with antiviral cover

## 6. Herpes zoster keratitis

| Acute epithelial | Nummular |
|---|---|
| 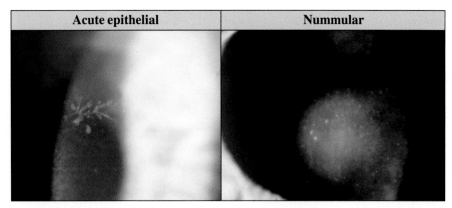 | |
| • Develops in about 50% within 2 days of rash | • Develops in about 30% within 10 days of rash |
| • Small, fine, dendritic or stellate epithelial lesions | • Multiple, fine, granular deposits just beneath Bowman membrane |
| • Tapered ends without bulbs | • Halo of stromal haze |
| • Resolves within a few days | • May become chronic |

*Treatment*  • Topical steroids, if appropriate

# CORNEAL DYSTROPHIES

1. **Anterior**
   - Cogan microcystic
   - Reis–Bücklers
   - Meesmann
   - Schnyder

2. **Stromal**
   - Lattice I, II, III
   - Granular I, II, III (Avellino)
   - Macular

3. **Posterior**
   - Fuchs endothelial
   - Posterior polymorphous

## 1. Anterior

**Cogan microcystic**

- Most common of all dystrophies
- Neither familial nor progressive
- Recurrent corneal erosions in about 10% of cases

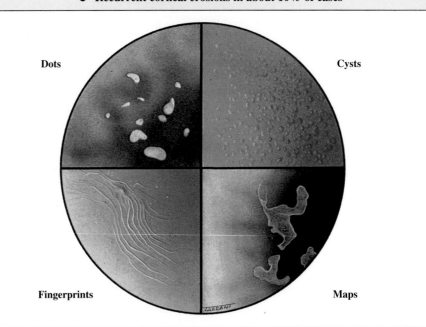

| | |
|---|---|
| Dots | Cysts |
| Fingerprints | Maps |

| Signs in isolation or combination ||
|---|---|
| **Dots** | **Microcysts** |

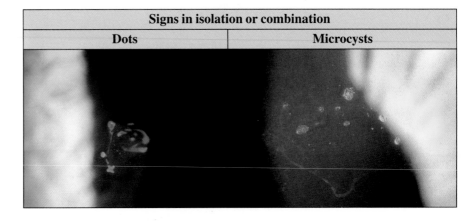

| Maps | Fingerprints |
|---|---|

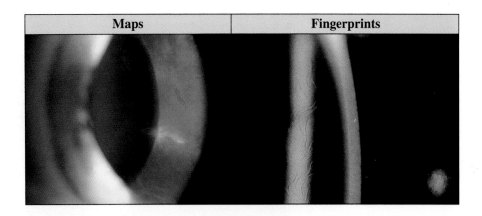

**Reis–Bücklers**

- Inheritance – autosomal dominant
- Onset – early childhood with recurrent corneal erosions

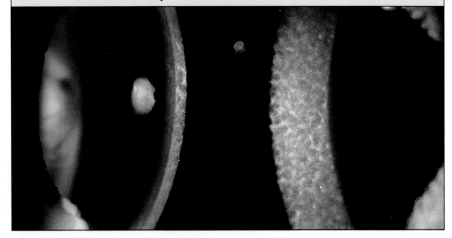

- Superficial polygonal opacities
- Honeycomb appearance

*Treatment*
- Keratoplasty if severe

**Meesmann**

- Inheritance – autosomal dominant
- Onset – first decade with mild visual symptoms

- Tiny, epithelial cysts, maximal centrally
- Clear on retroillumination
- Grey on direct illumination

*Treatment*
- Not required

**Schnyder**

- Inheritance – autosomal dominant
- Onset – second decade with visual impairment

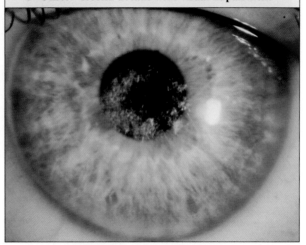

- Subepithelial 'crystalline' opacities

*Treatment*
- Excimer laser keratectomy

## 2. Stromal

- Inheritance – autosomal dominant
- Onset – late first decade with recurrent corneal erosions

**Lattice I**

**Progression**

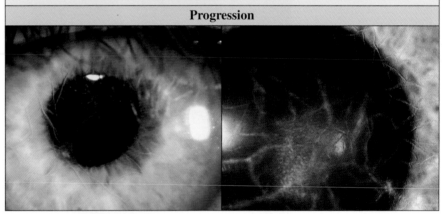

- Fine, spidery, branching lines within stroma
- Later general haze may submerge lesions

*Treatment*
- Penetrating keratoplasty if severe

**Lattice II**

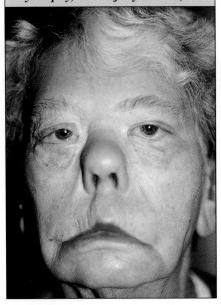

*(Familial amyloidosis with lattice dystrophy, Meretoja syndrome)*

*Inheritance*
- **Autosomal dominant**

*Onset*
- **Middle age with progressive facial palsy and lattice dystrophy identical to type I**

*Systemic features*
- **Cranial and peripheral neuropathy**
- **Skin laxity**
- **Renal and cardiac failure**

*Treatment*    • **Penetrating keratoplasty if severe**

**Lattice III**

- **Inheritance – autosomal dominant**
- **Onset – fourth decade**

- **Thick, ropey lines and minimal intervening haze**
- **May be asymmetrical and initially unilateral**

*Treatment*    • **Penetrating keratoplasty if severe**

**Granular I**

- Inheritance – autosomal dominant
- Onset – first decade with recurrent corneal erosions

**Progression**

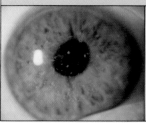 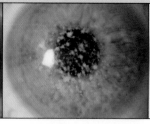 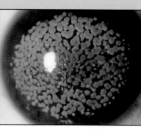

- Initial superficial and central crumb-like opacities
- Later deeper and peripheral spread but limbus spared
- Eventual confluence

*Treatment*

- Penetrating keratoplasty if severe

**Granular II**

- Inheritance – autosomal dominant
- Onset – fourth or fifth decade with mild recurrent erosions

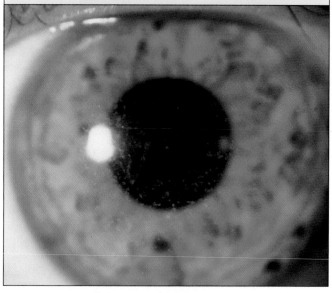

- Superficial, discrete crumb-like opacities

*Treatment*

- Penetrating keratoplasty if severe

**Granular III (Avellino)**

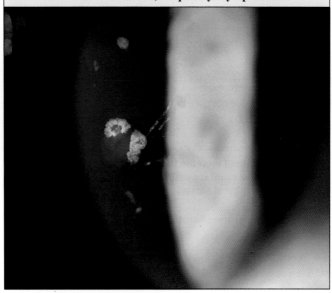

- Inheritance – autosomal dominant
- Onset – late in life; frequently asymptomatic

- Few, superficial, discrete, ring-shaped lesions
- Increase in density and size with time

*Treatment*

- Not required

**Macular**

- Inheritance – autosomal recessive
- Onset – second decade with painless visual loss

**Progression**

| | | |
|---|---|---|
| • Initial dense, poorly delineated opacities | • Later generalized opacification | • Thinning |

*Treatment*

- Penetrating keratoplasty

## 3. Posterior

**Fuchs endothelial**

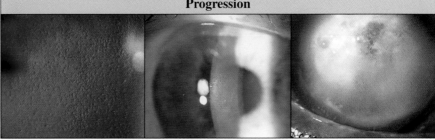

- Inheritance – occasionally autosomal dominant
- Onset – old age

### Progression

- Gradual increase in cornea guttata with peripheral spread
- Later central stromal oedema
- Eventually bullous keratopathy

*Treatment*

- Penetrating keratoplasty if advanced

**Posterior polymorphous**

- Inheritance – usually autosomal dominant
- Onset – difficult to determine because asymptomatic

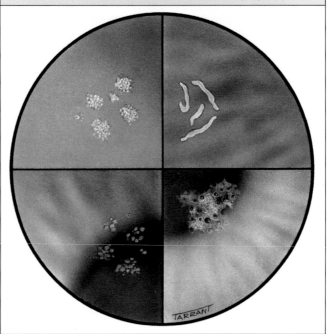

- Subtle, vesicular, geographic, or band-like lesions
- Frequently asymmetrical

*Treatment*

- Not required

# CORNEAL ECTASIAS

1.  **Keratoconus**

2.  **Keratoglobus**

3.  **Pellucid marginal degeneration**

## 1. Keratoconus

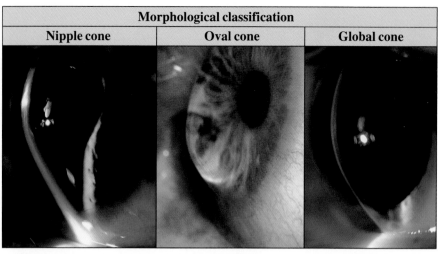

| Morphological classification | | |
|---|---|---|
| **Nipple cone** | **Oval cone** | **Global cone** |
| • Small and steep curvature | • Larger and ellipsoidal | • Largest |

| Signs | | |
|---|---|---|
| **Oil droplet reflex** | **Vogt striae** | **Prominent corneal nerves** |
| **Fleischer ring and scarring** | **Bulging of lower lids on downgaze** | **Acute hydrops** |
| | • Munson sign | |

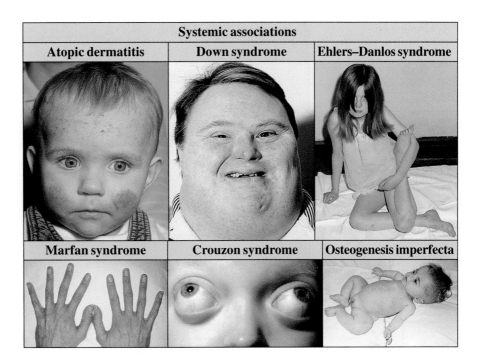

| Systemic associations | | |
|---|---|---|
| **Atopic dermatitis** | **Down syndrome** | **Ehlers–Danlos syndrome** |
| **Marfan syndrome** | **Crouzon syndrome** | **Osteogenesis imperfecta** |

## 2. Keratoglobus

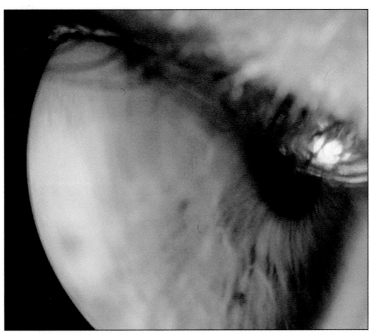

- Onset usually at birth
- Bilateral protrusion and thinning of entire cornea
- Associations – Leber congenital amaurosis and blue sclera

## 3. Pellucid marginal degeneration

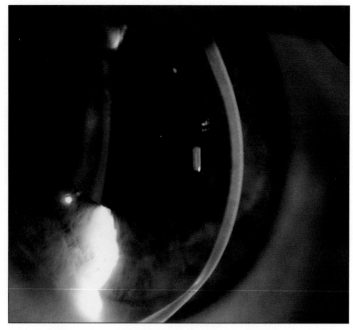

- Onset between 20 and 40 years
- Bilateral crescent-shaped inferior corneal thinning

# EPISCLERITIS AND SCLERITIS

1. **Episcleritis**
   - Simple
   - Nodular

2. **Anterior scleritis**
   - Non-necrotizing diffuse
   - Non-necrotizing nodular
   - Necrotizing with inflammation
   - Necrotizing without inflammation (scleromalacia perforans)

3. **Posterior scleritis**

| Applied anatomy of vascular coats | | |
|---|---|---|
| **Normal** | **Episcleritis** | **Scleritis** |
| 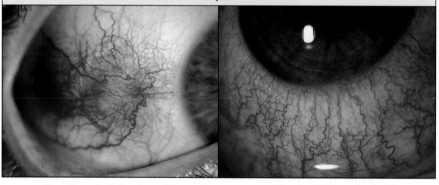 | | |
| • Radial superficial episcleral vessels<br>• Deep vascular plexus adjacent to sclera | • Maximal congestion of episcleral vessels | • Maximal congestion of deep vascular plexus<br>• Slight congestion of episcleral vessels |

## 1. Episcleritis

**Simple**

- Common, benign, self-limiting but frequently recurrent
- Typically affects young adults
- Seldom associated with a systemic disorder

- Simple sectorial episcleritis
- Simple diffuse episcleritis

*Treatment*

- Topical steroids
- Oral flurbiprofen (100 mg tid) if unresponsive

**Nodular**

- Less common than simple episcleritis
- May take longer to resolve
- Treatment – similar to simple episcleritis

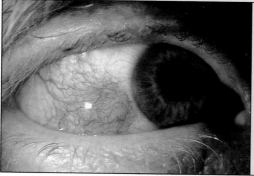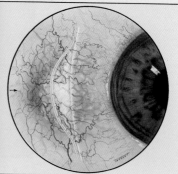

- Localized nodule which can be moved over sclera
- Deep scleral part of slit-beam not displaced

**2. Anterior scleritis**

## CAUSES AND SYSTEMIC ASSOCIATIONS OF SCLERITIS

1. Rheumatoid arthritis
2. Connective tissue disorders
   - Wegener granulomatosis
   - Polyarteritis nodosa
   - Systemic lupus erythematosus
3. Miscellaneous
   - Relapsing polychondritis
   - Herpes zoster ophthalmicus
   - Surgically induced

**Non-necrotizing diffuse**

- Relatively benign – does not progress to necrosis
- Widespread scleral and episcleral injection

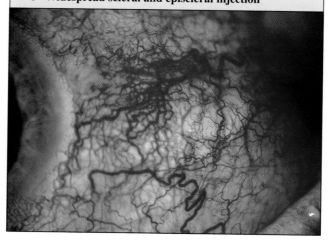

*Treatment*
- Oral non-steroidal anti-inflammatory drugs
- Oral steroids if unresponsive

**Non-necrotizing nodular**

- ● More serious than diffuse scleritis

- ● On cursory examination resembles nodular episcleritis
- ● Scleral nodule cannot be moved over underlying tissue

*Treatment*
- ● Similar to non-necrotizing diffuse scleritis

**Necrotizing with inflammation**

- ● Painful and most severe type
- ● Complications – uveitis, keratitis, cataract and glaucoma

**Progression**

- ● Avascular patches
- ● Scleral necrosis and visibility of uvea
- ● Spread and coalescence of necrosis

*Treatment Options*
- ● Oral steroids
- ● Immunosuppressive agents (cyclophosphamide, azathioprine, cyclosporin)
- ● Combined intravenous steroids and cyclophosphamide if unresponsive

**Necrotizing without inflammation (scleromalacia perforans)**

- Associated with rheumatoid arthritis
- Asymptomatic and untreatable

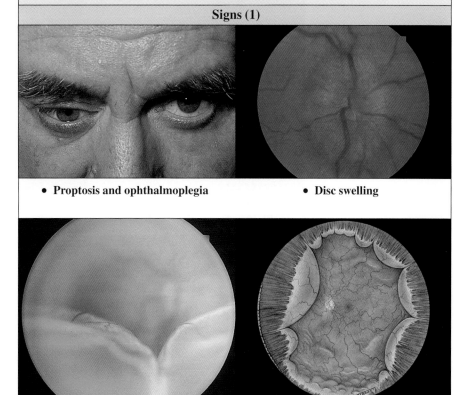

- Progressive scleral thinning with exposure of underlying uvea

## 3. Posterior scleritis

- About 20% of all cases of scleritis
- About 30% of patients have systemic disease
- Treatment similar to necrotizing scleritis with inflammation

### Signs (1)

- Proptosis and ophthalmoplegia
- Disc swelling

- Exudative retinal detachment
- Ring choroidal detachment

## Signs (2)

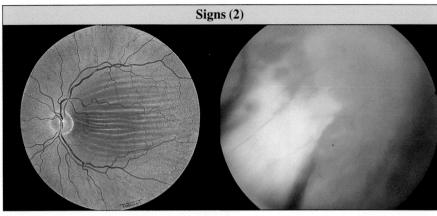

- Choroidal folds
- Subretinal exudation

## Imaging

| Ultrasound | Axial CT |
|---|---|

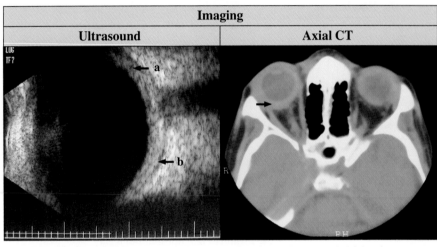

- Thickening of posterior sclera (a)
- Fluid in Tenon space – 'T' sign (b)

- Posterior scleral thickening

# ACQUIRED CATARACT

1. **Classification of age-related cataract**
   - **Morphological**
   - **According to maturity**

2. **Other causes of cataract**
   - **Diabetes**
   - **Myotonic dystrophy**
   - **Atopic dermatitis**
   - **Trauma**
   - **Drugs**
   - **Secondary (complicated)**

3. **Surgery**
   - **Large incision extracapsular**
   - **Phacoemulsification**

## 1. Classification of age-related cataract

### CLASSIFICATION OF AGE-RELATED CATARACT ACCORDING TO MORPHOLOGY

1. Subcapsular
   - Anterior
   - Posterior
2. Nuclear
3. Cortical
4. Christmas tree

| Subcapsular | |
| --- | --- |
| Anterior | Posterior |

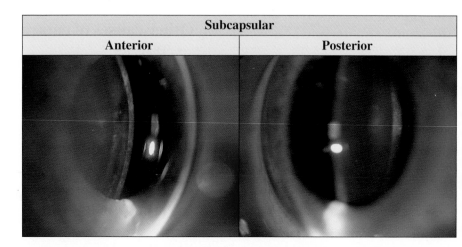

**Progression of nuclear cataract**

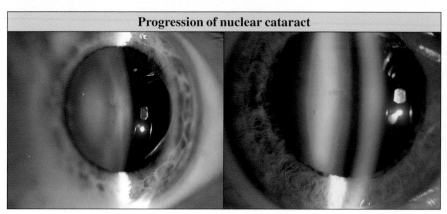

- Exaggeration of normal nuclear ageing change
- Causes increasing myopia

- Increasing nuclear opacification
- Initially yellow then brown

## Progression of nuclear cataract

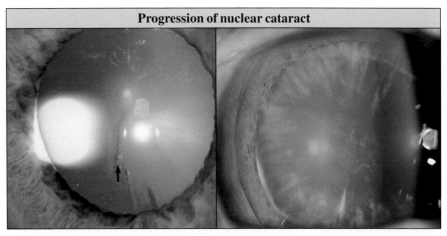

- Initially vacuoles and clefts
- Progressive radial spoke-like opacities

## Christmas tree

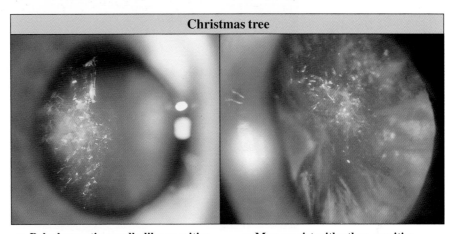

- Polychromatic, needle-like opacities
- May coexist with other opacities

**According to maturity**

| Immature | Mature |
| --- | --- |

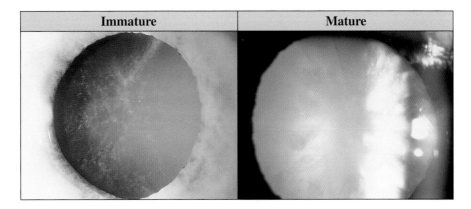

| Hypermature | Morgagnian |
| --- | --- |

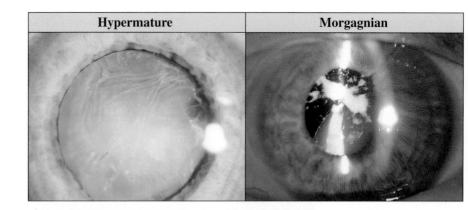

## 2. Other causes of cataract

### Diabetes

| Juvenile | Adult |
| --- | --- |

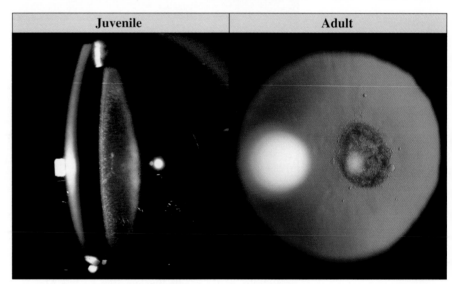

- White punctate or snowflake posterior or anterior opacities
- May mature within few days

- Cortical and subcapsular opacities
- May progress more quickly than in non-diabetics

**Myotonic dystrophy**

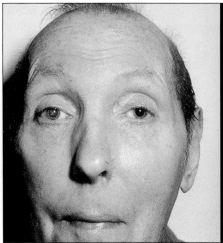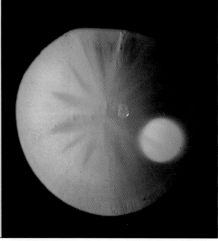

- Myotonic facies
- Frontal balding

- Stellate posterior subcapsular opacity
- 90% of patients after age 20 years
- No visual problem until age 40 years

**Atopic dermatitis**

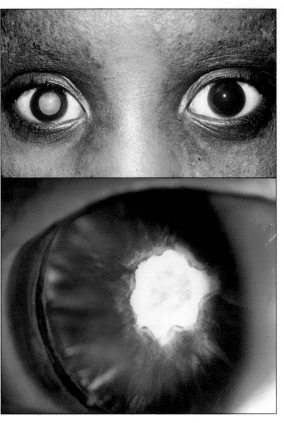

- Cataract develops in 10% of cases between 15 and 30 years
- Bilateral in 70%
- Frequently becomes mature

- Anterior subcapsular plaque (shield cataract)
- Wrinkles in anterior capsule

**Trauma**

| Concussion |
|---|

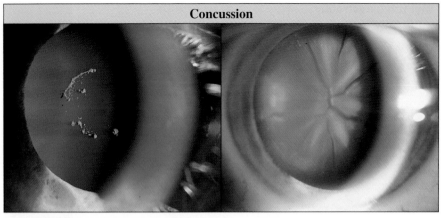

- Vossius ring from imprinting of iris pigment
- Flower-shaped

| Penetration |
|---|

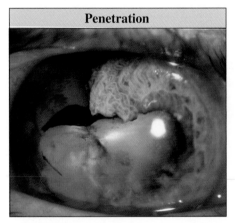

*Other causes*
- Ionizing radiation
- Electric shock
- Lightning

**Drugs**

| Systemic or topical steroids | Chlorpromazine |
|---|---|
| Initially posterior subcapsular | Central, anterior capsular granules |

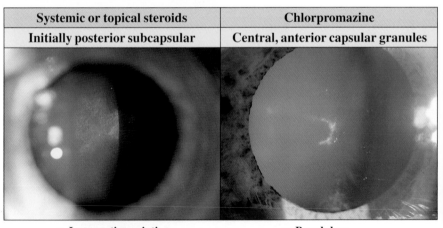

*Other drugs*
- Long-acting miotics
- Amiodarone
- Busulphan

**Secondary (complicated)**

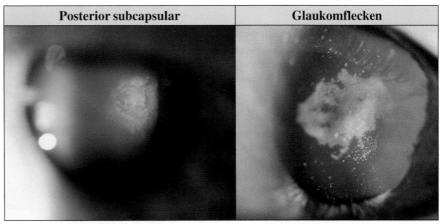

| Posterior subcapsular | Glaukomflecken |
|---|---|
| • Chronic anterior uveitis<br>• High myopia<br>• Hereditary fundus dystrophies | • Follows acute angle-closure glaucoma<br>• Central, anterior subcapsular opacities |

## 3. Surgery

**Large incision extracapsular extraction**

1. Anterior capsulotomy

2. Completion of incision

3. Expression of nucleus

4. Cortical cleanup

5. Care not to aspirate posterior capsule accidentally

6. Polishing of posterior capsule, if appropriate

7. Injection of viscoelastic substance

8. Grasping of IOL and coating with viscoelastic substance

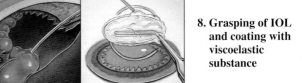

9. Insertion of
   inferior haptic
   and optic

10. Insertion of
    superior haptic

11. Placement of
    haptics into
    capsular bag
    and not into
    ciliary sulcus

12. Dialling of IOL
    into horizontal
    position

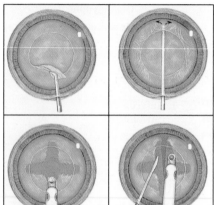

**Phacoemulsification**

1. Capsulorrhexis

2. Hydrodissection

3. Sculpting of
   nucleus

4. Cracking of
   nucleus

5. Emulsification of
   each quadrant

6. Cortical cleanup
   and insertion of
   IOL

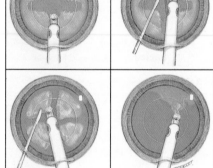

# CONGENITAL CATARACT

1. **Important facts**

2. **Classification**

3. **Causes**
   - In healthy neonate
   - In unwell neonate

## 1. Important facts

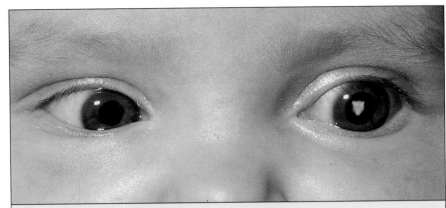

- 33% – idiopathic – may be unilateral or bilateral
- 33% – inherited – usually bilateral
- 33% – associated with systemic disease – usually bilateral
- Other ocular anomalies present in 50%

## 2. Classification

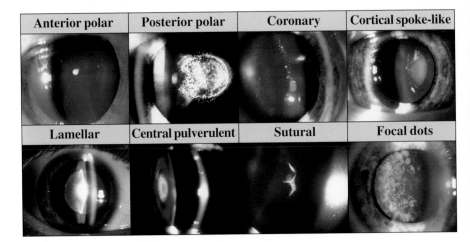

| Anterior polar | Posterior polar | Coronary | Cortical spoke-like |
| --- | --- | --- | --- |

| Lamellar | Central pulverulent | Sutural | Focal dots |
| --- | --- | --- | --- |

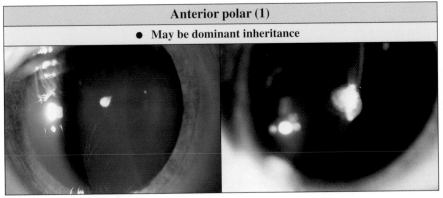

**Anterior polar (1)**

- May be dominant inheritance

- Capsular                    - Pyramid

## Anterior polar (2)

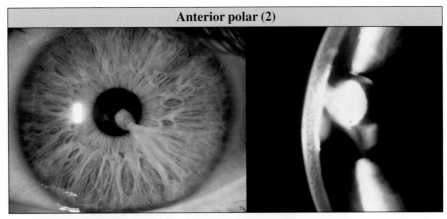

- **With persistent pupillary membrane**
- **With Peters anomaly**

## Posterior polar

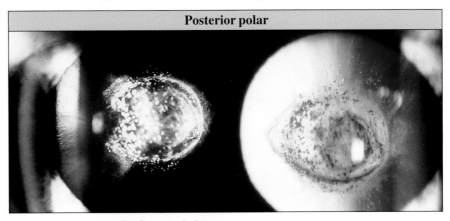

*Ocular associations*
- **Persistent hyaloid remnants**
- **Posterior lenticonus**
- **Persistent hyperplastic primary vitreous**

## Coronary (supranuclear)

- Usually sporadic

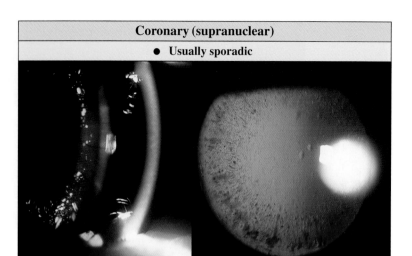

- Round opacities in deep cortex
- Surround nucleus like a crown

## Cortical spoke-like

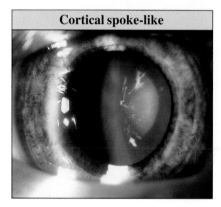

*Systemic associations*
- Fabry disease
- Mannosidosis

## Lamellar

- Usually dominant inheritance

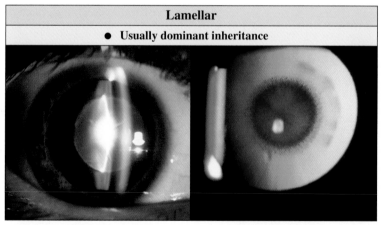

- Round central shell-like opacity surrounding clear nucleus
- May have riders

*Systemic associations*
- Galactosaemia
- Hypoglycaemia
- Hypocalcaemia

## Central pulverulent

● **Dominant inheritance**

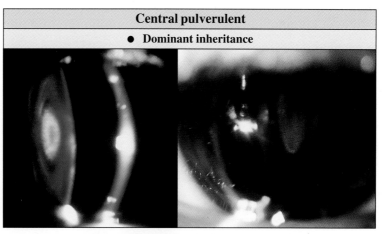

- Spheroidal opacity within nucleus
- Relatively clear centre
- Non-progressive

## Sutural

● **Usually X-linked inheritance**

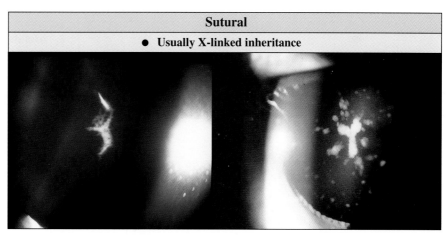

- Opacity follows shape of Y suture

## Focal dot opacities

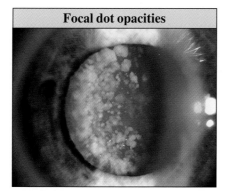

- Blue dot cortical opacities
- Common and innocuous
- May coexist with other opacities

### 3. Causes

**In healthy neonate**

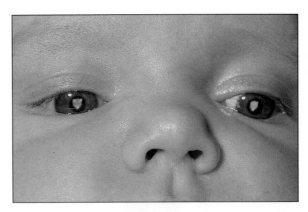

1. **Hereditary (usually dominant)**
2. **Idiopathic**
3. **With ocular anomalies**
   - **PHPV**
   - **Aniridia**
   - **Coloboma**
   - **Microphthalmos**
   - **Buphthalmos**

**In unwell neonate**

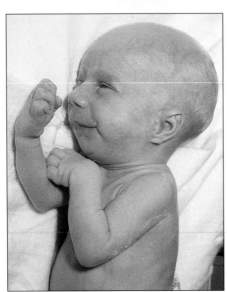

1. **Intrauterine infections**
   - **Rubella**
   - **Toxoplasmosis**
   - **Cytomegalovirus**
   - **Varicella**

2. **Metabolic disorders**
   - **Galactosaemia**
   - **Hypoglycaemia**
   - **Hypocalcaemia**
   - **Lowe syndrome**

# COMPLICATIONS OF CATARACT SURGERY

1. **Operative complications**
   - **Vitreous loss**
   - **Posterior loss of lens fragments**
   - **Suprachoroidal (expulsive) haemorrhage**

2. **Early postoperative complications**
   - **Iris prolapse**
   - **Striate keratopathy**
   - **Acute bacterial endophthalmitis**

3. **Late postoperative complications**
   - **Capsular opacification**
   - **Implant displacement**
   - **Corneal decompensation**
   - **Retinal detachment**
   - **Chronic bacterial endophthalmitis**

## 1. Operative complications

**Vitreous loss**

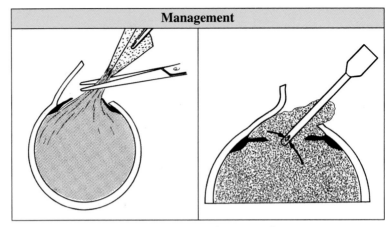

Management

- Sponge or automated anterior vitrectomy
- Insertion of PC-IOL if adequate capsular support present

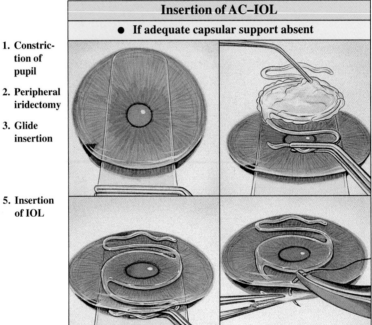

Insertion of AC–IOL

- If adequate capsular support absent

1. Constriction of pupil

2. Peripheral iridectomy

3. Glide insertion

4. Coating of IOL with viscoelastic substance

5. Insertion of IOL

6. Suturing of incision

**Posterior loss of lens fragments**

| Management |
| --- |
| ● **Fragments consisting of 25% or more of lens should be removed** |

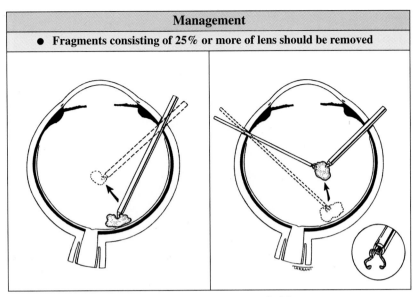

● **Pars plana vitrectomy and removal of fragment**

**Suprachoroidal (expulsive) haemorrhage**

| Management |
| --- |
| ● **Close incision and administer hyperosmotic agent** |
| **Subsequent treatment after 7–14 days** |

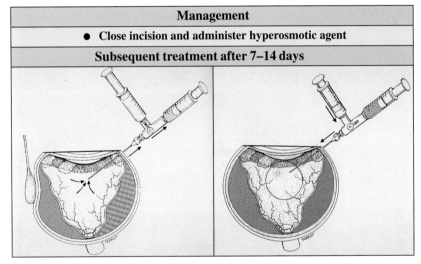

● **Drain blood**
● **Pars plana vitrectomy**
● **Air–fluid exchange**

## 2. Early postoperative complications

**Iris prolapse**

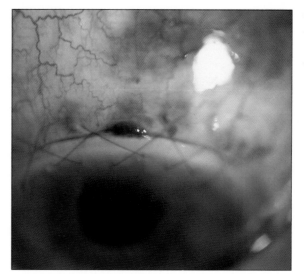

*Cause*

- Usually inadequate suturing of incision
- Most frequently follows inappropriate management of vitreous loss

*Treatment*

- Excise prolapsed iris tissue
- Resuture incision

**Striate keratopathy**

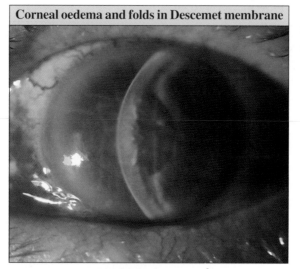

Corneal oedema and folds in Descemet membrane

*Cause*

- Damage to endothelium during surgery

*Treatment*

- Most cases resolve within a few days
- Occasionally persistent cases may require penetrating keratoplasty

**Acute bacterial endophthalmitis**

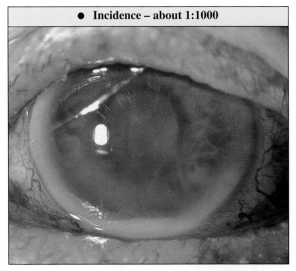

● Incidence – about 1:1000

*Common causative organisms*
- *Staph. epidermidis*
- *Staph. aureus*
- *Pseudomonas* sp.

*Source of infection*
- Patient's own external bacterial flora is most frequent culprit
- Contaminated solutions and instruments
- Environmental flora including that of surgeon and operating room personnel

**Preoperative prophylaxis**

**Treatment of pre-existing infections**

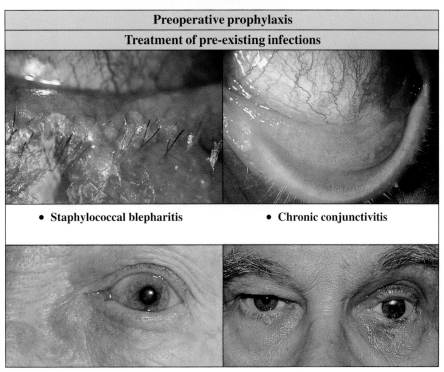

- Staphylococcal blepharitis
- Chronic conjunctivitis
- Chronic dacryocystitis
- Infected socket

## Peroperative prophylaxis

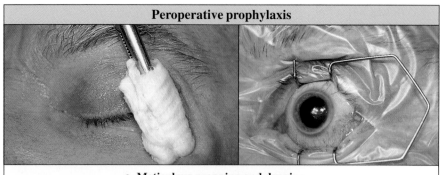

- Meticulous prepping and draping

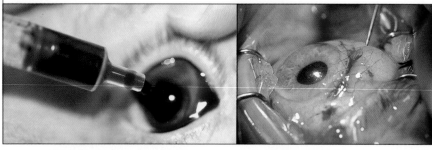

- Instillation of povidone-iodine
- Postoperative injection of antibiotics

## Signs of severe endophthalmitis

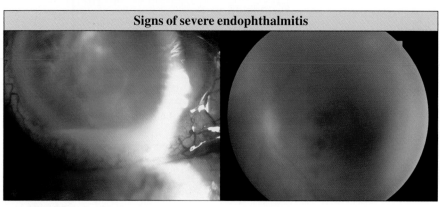

- Pain and marked visual loss
- Corneal haze, fibrinous exudate and hypopyon

- Absent or poor red reflex
- Inability to visualize fundus with indirect ophthalmoscope

| Signs of mild endophthalmitis |
| --- |

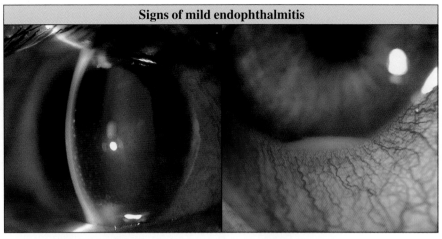

- Mild pain and visual loss
- Anterior chamber cells

- Small hypopyon
- Fundus visible with indirect ophthalmoscope

| Differential diagnosis of endophthalmitis | |
| --- | --- |
| Uveitis associated with retained lens material | Sterile fibrinous reaction |

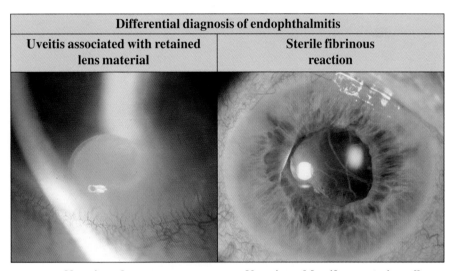

- No pain or hypopyon

- No pain and few if any anterior cells
- Posterior synechiae may develop

## MANAGEMENT OF ACUTE ENDOPHTHALMITIS

1. Preparation of intravitreal injections
2. Identification of causative organisms
   - Aqueous samples
   - Vitreous samples
3. Intravitreal injections of antibiotics
4. Vitrectomy – only if VA is PL
5. Subsequent treatment

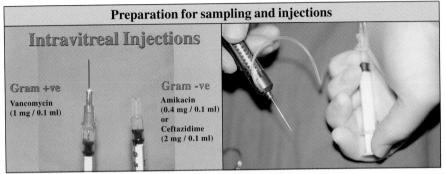

**Preparation for sampling and injections**

**Intravitreal Injections**

Gram +ve

Vancomycin
(1 mg / 0.1 ml)

Gram -ve

Amikacin
(0.4 mg / 0.1 ml)
or
Ceftazidime
(2 mg / 0.1 ml)

- Antibiotics
- Mini vitrector

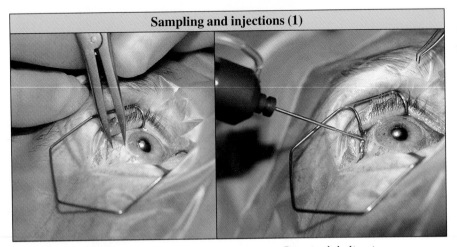

**Sampling and injections (1)**

- Make partial-thickness sclerotomy 3 mm behind limbus
- Insert mini vitrector

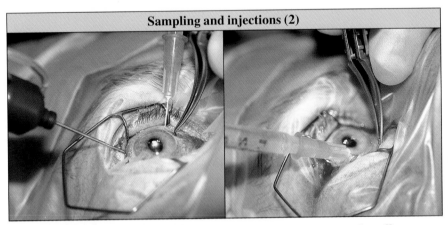

**Sampling and injections (2)**

- Insert needle attached to syringe containing antibiotics
- Aspirate 0.3 ml with vitrector
- Give first injection of antibiotics
- Disconnect syringe from needle
- Give second injection

- Remove vitrector and needle
- Inject subconjunctival antibiotics

## SUBSEQUENT TREATMENT

1. **Periocular injections**
   - Vancomycin 25 mg with ceftazidime 100 mg or gentamicin 20 mg with cefuroxime 125 mg
   - Betamethasone 4 mg (1 ml)
2. **Topical therapy**
   - Fortified gentamicin 15 mg/ml and vancomycin 50 mg/ml drops
   - Dexamethasone 0.1%
3. **Systemic therapy**
   - Antibiotics are not beneficial
   - Steroids only in very severe cases

## 3. Late postoperative complications

**Capsular opacification**

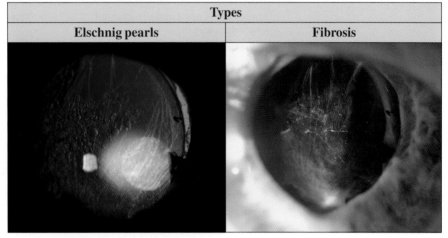

| Types | |
|---|---|
| **Elschnig pearls** | **Fibrosis** |

- Proliferation of lens epithelium
- Occurs after 3–5 years

- Usually occurs within 2–6 months
- May involve remnants of anterior capsule and cause phimosis

### Treatment

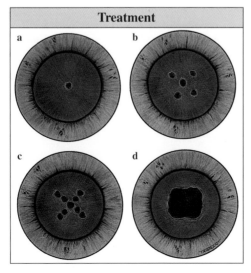

*Nd:YAG laser capsulotomy*
- Accurate focusing is vital
- Apply series of punctures in cruciate pattern (a–c)
- 3 mm opening is adequate (d)

*Potential complications*
- Damage to implant
- Cystoid macular oedema – uncommon
- Retinal detachment – rare except in high myopes

**Implant displacement**

| Decentration | Optic capture |
|---|---|

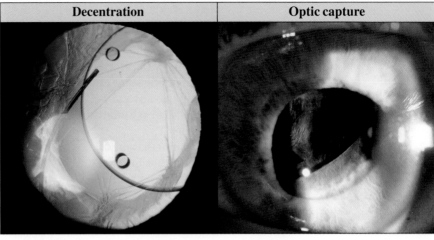

- May occur if one haptic is inserted into sulcus and other into bag
- Remove and replace if severe

- Reposition may be necessary

**Corneal decompensation**

| Predispositions | Treatment |
|---|---|

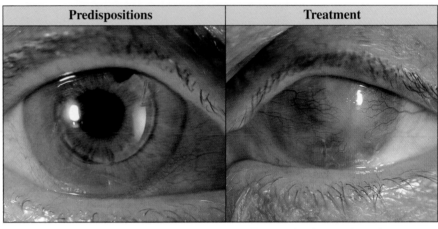

- Anterior chamber implant
- Fuchs endothelial dystrophy

- Penetrating keratoplasty in severe cases
- Guarded visual prognosis because of frequently associated CMO

**Retinal detachment**

| Risk factors | |
|---|---|
| **Disruption of posterior capsule** | **Lattice degeneration** |

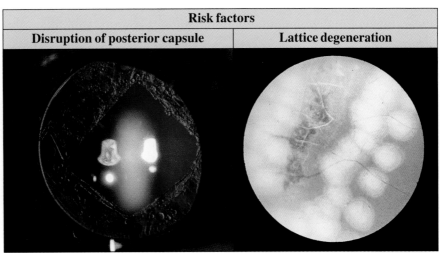

- Intraoperative vitreous loss
- Laser capsulotomy, particularly in high myopia

- Treat prophylactically before or soon after surgery

**Chronic bacterial endophthalmitis**

| Signs | |
|---|---|

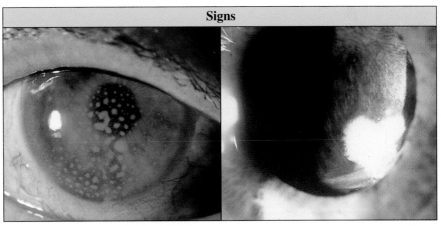

- Late onset, persistent, low-grade uveitis – may be granulomatous
- Commonly caused by *Propionibacterium acnes* or *Staph. epidermidis*

- Low virulence organisms trapped in capsular bag
- White plaque on posterior capsule

## Treatment

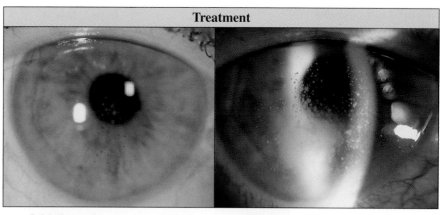

- Initially good response to topical steroids

- Recurrence after cessation of treatment
- Inject intravitreal vancomycin
- Remove IOL and capsular bag if unresponsive

# ECTOPIA LENTIS

1. **Acquired**

2. **Isolated familial**

3. **Associated with systemic disorders**
   - Marfan syndrome
   - Weill–Marchesani syndrome
   - Homocystinuria

## 1. Acquired

| Trauma | Stretched zonules |
|---|---|
| 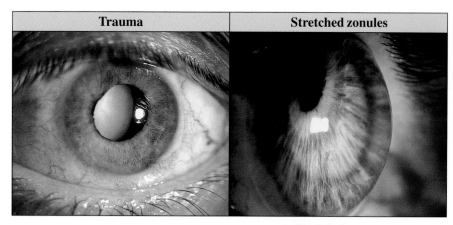 | |

- Buphthalmos
- Megalocornea

| Anterior uveal tumours | Degenerate eye |
|---|---|
| 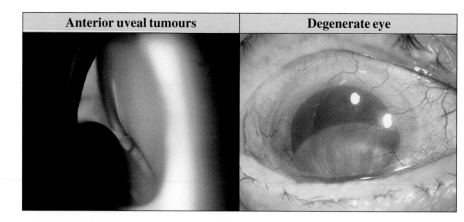 | |

## 2. Isolated familial

**Autosomal recessive ectopia lentis**

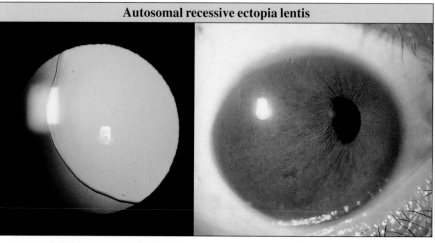

- Pupil may be normal
- Pupil may be displaced in opposite direction (ectopia lentis et pupillae)

## 3. Associated with systemic disorders

**Marfan syndrome**

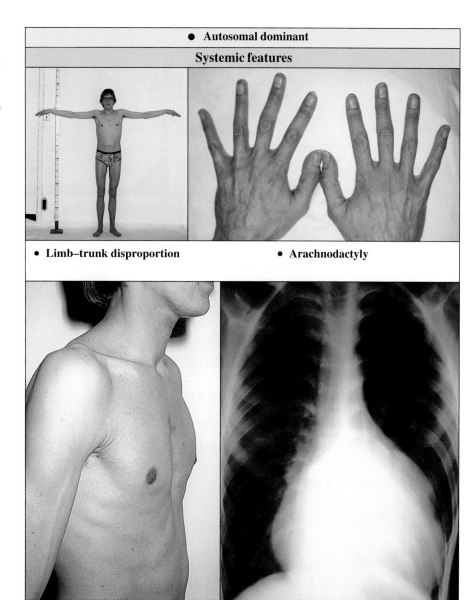

- Autosomal dominant

**Systemic features**

- Limb–trunk disproportion
- Arachnodactyly

- Pectus excavatum
- High-arched palate

- Aortic dilatation, dissection and regurgitation
- Mitral valve prolapse

| Ocular features | | |
|---|---|---|
| Lens | Retinal detachment | |
| 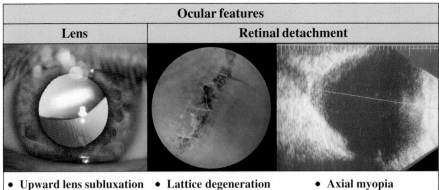 | | |
| • Upward lens subluxation<br>• Zonule usually intact | • Lattice degeneration | • Axial myopia |
| Angle anomaly and glaucoma | Cornea plana | Blue sclera |

**Weill–Marchesani syndrome**

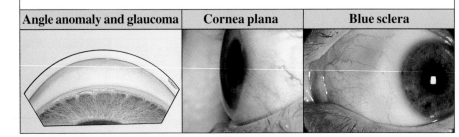

| • Autosomal recessive | |
|---|---|
| Systemic features | Ocular features |

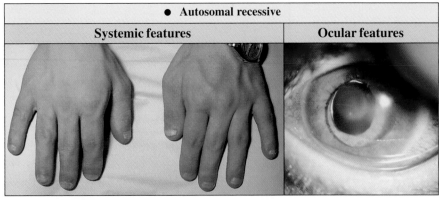

- Short stature
- Short stubby fingers (brachydactyly)
- Mental handicap

- Microspherophakia
- Usually anterior lens subluxation
- Angle anomaly and glaucoma

**Homocystinuria**

- Autosomal recessive
- Defect in cystathione beta-synthetase

| Systemic features | Ocular features |
|---|---|
| 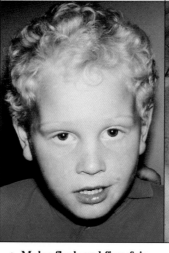 | 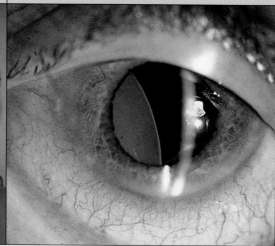 |

- Malar flush and fine, fair hair
- Marfanoid habitus
- Increased platelet stickiness
- Mental handicap

- Downward lens subluxation
- Disintegration of zonule

## TREATMENT OPTIONS FOR ECTOPIA LENTIS

1. Spectacle correction
    - For induced astigmatism
    - For aphakic portion
2. Nd:YAG laser zonulysis to displace lens out of visual axis
3. Surgical removal
    - Associated cataract
    - Lens-induced glaucoma
    - Endothelial touch
    - When other methods are inappropriate

# INTRODUCTION TO GLAUCOMA

1. **Aqueous outflow**
   - Anatomy
   - Physiology

2. **Classification of secondary glaucomas**

3. **Tonometers**

4. **Gonioscopy**

5. **Anatomy of retinal nerve fibres**

6. **Optic nerve head**

7. **Humphrey perimetry**

## 1. Aqueous outflow

**Anatomy**

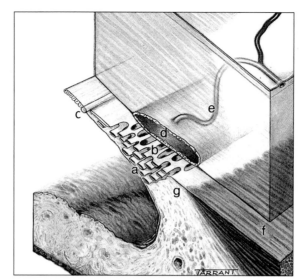

- Uveal meshwork (a)
- Corneoscleral meshwork (b)
- Schwalbe line (c)
- Schlemm canal (d)
- Collector channels (e)
- Longitudinal muscle of ciliary body (f)
- Scleral spur (g)

**Physiology**

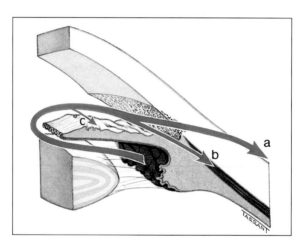

- Conventional outflow (a)
- Uveoscleral outflow (b)
- Iris outflow (c)

## 2. Classification of secondary glaucomas

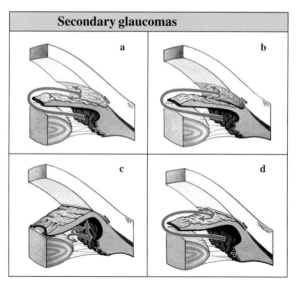

**Secondary glaucomas**

*Open-angle*
- *Pre-trabecular* – membrane over trabeculum (a)
- *Trabecular* – 'clogging up' of trabeculum (b)

*Angle-closure*
- *With pupil block* – seclusio pupillae and iris bombé (c)
- *Without pupil block* – peripheral anterior synechiae (d)

## 3. Tonometers

| Goldmann | Perkins |
|---|---|

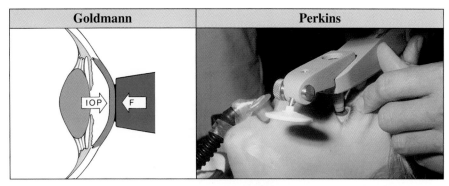

- Contact applanation
- Portable contact applanation

| Schiotz | Air-puff |
|---|---|

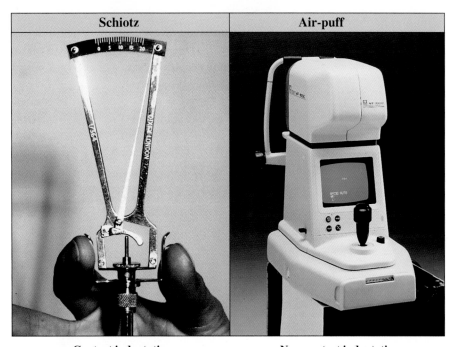

- Contact indentation
- Non-contact indentation

| Pulsair 2000 (Keeler) | Tono-Pen |
|---|---|

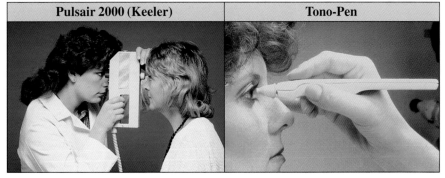

- Portable non-contact applanation
- Portable contact applanation

## 4. Gonioscopy

| Goniolenses | |
| --- | --- |
| **Goldmann** | **Zeiss** |

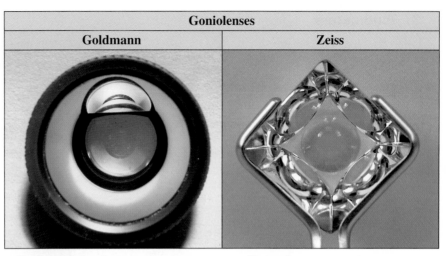

- Single or triple mirror
- Contact surface diameter 12 mm
- Coupling substance required
- Suitable for ALT
- Not suitable for indentation gonioscopy

- Four mirror
- Contact surface diameter 9 mm
- Coupling substance not required
- Not suitable for ALT
- Suitable for indentation gonioscopy

| Indentation gonioscopy |
| --- |
| ● Differentiates 'appositional' from 'synechial' angle closure |

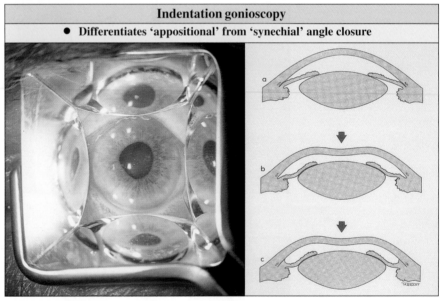

- Press Zeiss lens posteriorly against cornea

- Aqueous is forced into periphery of anterior chamber

| Indentation in iridocorneal contact | |
|---|---|
| **During indentation** | **Before indentation** |

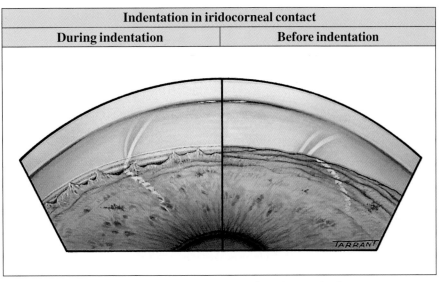

| | |
|---|---|
| • Part of angle is forced open | • Complete angle closure |
| • Part of angle remains closed by PAS | • Apex of corneal wedge not visible |

| Angle structures |
|---|

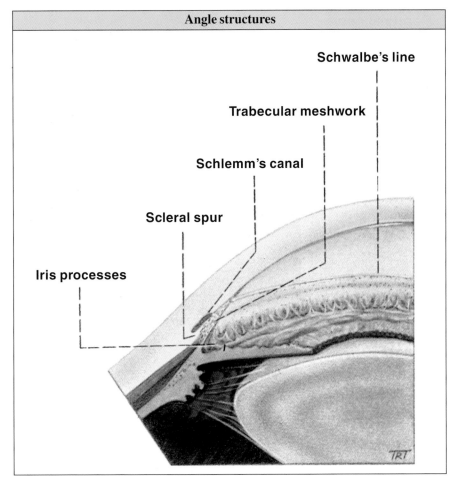

Schwalbe's line

Trabecular meshwork

Schlemm's canal

Scleral spur

Iris processes

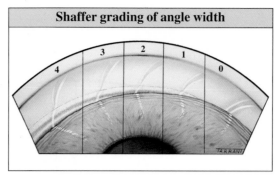

**Shaffer grading of angle width**

*Grade 4 (35–45°)*
- Ciliary body easily visible

*Grade 3 (25–35°)*
- At least scleral spur visible

*Grade 2 (20°)*
- Only trabeculum visible
- Angle closure possible but unlikely

*Grade 1 (10°)*
- Only Schwalbe line and perhaps top of trabeculum visible
- High risk of angle closure

*Grade 0 (0°)*
- Iridocorneal contact present
- Apex of corneal wedge not visible
- Use indentation gonioscopy

## 5. Anatomy of retinal nerve fibres

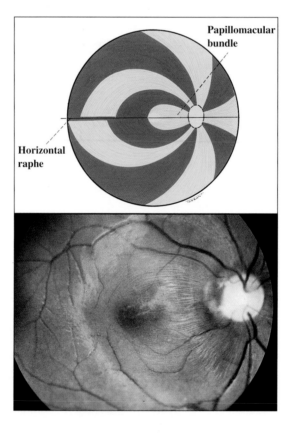

## 6. Optic nerve head

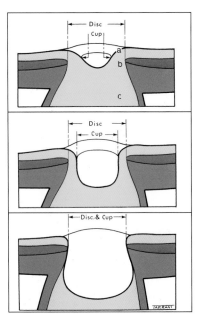

*Small physiological cup*
- Nerve fibre layer (a)
- Prelaminar layer (b)
- Laminar layer (c)

*Large physiological cup*
- Normal vertical cup–disc ratio is 0.3 or less
- 2% of population have cup–disc ratio > 0.7
- Asymmetry of 0.2 or more is suspicious

*Total glaucomatous cupping*

### Types of physiological excavation

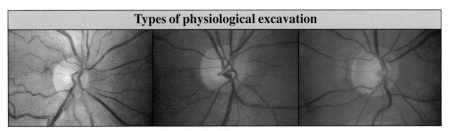

- Small dimple central cup
- Larger and deeper punched-out central cup
- Cup with sloping temporal wall

### Pallor and cupping

- Pallor – maximal area of colour contrast
- Cupping – bending of small blood vessels crossing disc

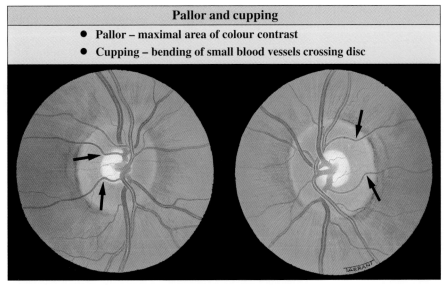

- Cupping and pallor correspond
- Cupping is greater than pallor

## 7. Humphrey perimetry

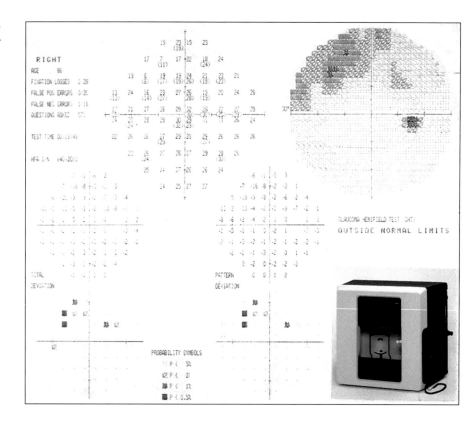

## RELIABILITY INDICES

1. **Fixation losses**
   - **Detected by presenting stimuli in blind spot**
2. **False positives**
   - **Stimulus accompanied by a sound**
   - **High score suggests a 'trigger happy' patient**
3. **False negatives**
   - **Failure to respond to a stimulus 9 dB brighter than previously seen at same location**
   - **High score indicates inattention, or advanced field loss**

## DEVIATIONS

1. Total
   - Upper numerical display shows difference (dB) between patient's results and age-matched normals
   - Lower graphic display shows these differences as grey scale
2. Pattern
   - Similar to total deviation
   - Adjusted for any generalized depression in overall field

## GLOBAL INDICES

1. Mean deviation (elevation or depression)
   - Deviation of patient's overall field from normal
   - $p$ values are $< 5\%$, $< 2\%$, $< 1\%$ and $< 0.5\%$
   - The lower the $p$ value the greater the significance
2. Pattern standard deviation
   - Departure of visual field from age-matched normals
3. Short-term fluctuation
   - Consistency of responses
   - 2 dB or less indicates reliable field
   - $> 3$ dB indicates either unreliable or damaged field
4. Corrected pattern standard deviation
   - Departure of overall shape of patient's hill of vision from age-matched normals

# PRIMARY OPEN-ANGLE GLAUCOMA

1.  **Definition and risk factors**

2.  **Theories of glaucomatous damage**

3.  **Optic disc cupping**

4.  **Visual field defects**

5.  **Medical therapy**

6.  **Laser trabeculoplasty**
    - Indications
    - Technique

7.  **Trabeculectomy**
    - Indications
    - Technique
    - Filtration blebs
    - Complications

## 1. Definition and risk factors

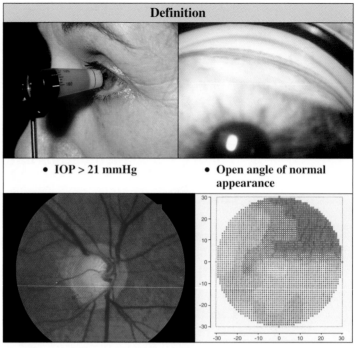

**Definition**

- IOP > 21 mmHg

- Open angle of normal appearance

- Glaucomatous disc damage

- Visual field loss

| RISK FACTORS |
| --- |
| 1. **Age** – most cases present after age 65 years<br>2. **Race** – more common, earlier onset and more severe in blacks<br>3. **Inheritance**<br>   • Level of IOP, outflow facility and disc size are inherited<br>   • Risk is increased × 2 if parent has POAG<br>   • Risk is increased × 4 if sibling has POAG<br>4. **Myopia** |

## 2. Theories of glaucoma-tous damage

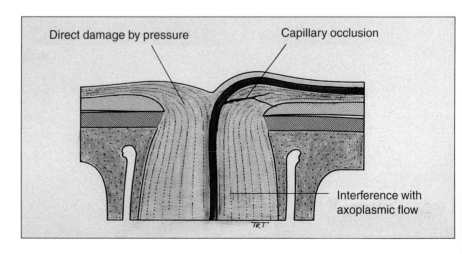

Direct damage by pressure

Capillary occlusion

Interference with axoplasmic flow

**3. Optic disc cupping**

**Localized cupping**

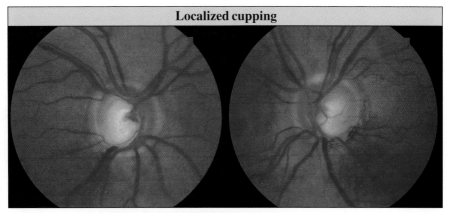

- Focal loss of nerve fibres
- Notching at superior or more commonly inferior poles
- Excavation becomes vertically oval
- Double angulation of blood vessels ('bayoneting sign')

**Concentric cupping**

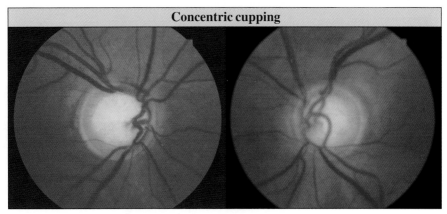

- Diffuse loss of nerve fibres
- Excavation enlarges concentrically

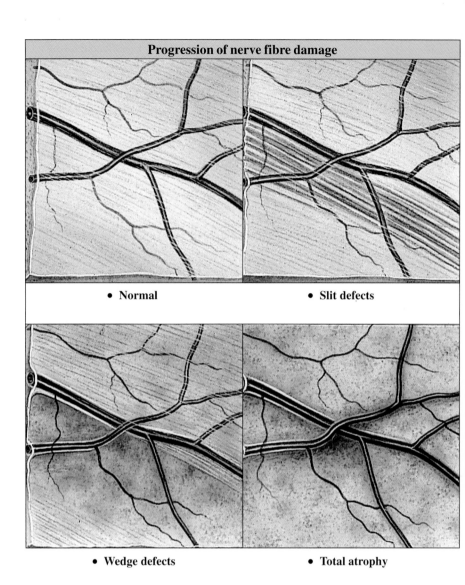

**Progression of nerve fibre damage**

- Normal
- Slit defects
- Wedge defects
- Total atrophy

## End-stage damage

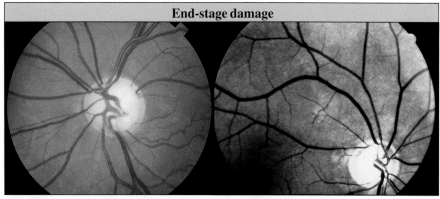

- All neural disc tissue is destroyed
- Disc is white and deeply excavated

- Atrophy of all retinal nerve fibres
- Striations are absent
- Blood vessels appear dark and sharply defined

## Progression of glaucomatous cupping

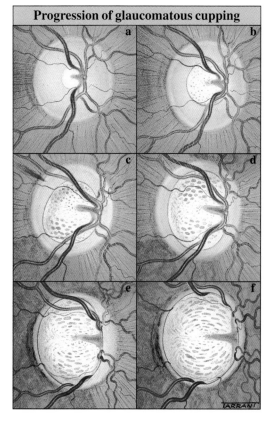

- Normal (c:d ratio 0.2) (a)

- Concentric enlargement (c:d ratio 0.5) (b)

- Inferior expansion with retinal nerve fibre loss (c)

- Superior expansion with retinal nerve fibre loss (d)

- Advanced cupping with nasal displacement of vessels (e)

- Total cupping with loss of all retinal nerve fibres (f)

## 4. Visual field defects

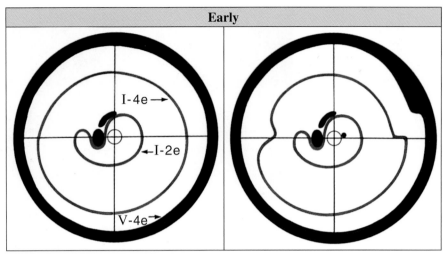

**Early**

- Small arcuate scotomas
- Tend to elongate circumferentially

- Isolated paracentral scotomas
- Nasal (Roenne) step

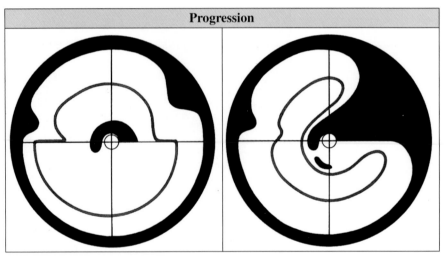

**Progression**

- Formation of arcuate defects
- Enlargement of nasal step
- Development of temporal wedge

- Peripheral breakthrough
- Appearance of fresh arcuate inferior defects

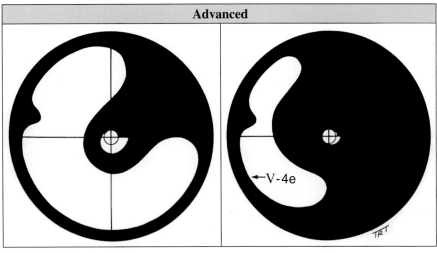

| **Advanced** |
|---|

| | |
|---|---|
| • Development of ring scotoma | • Peripheral and central spread |
| • Residual central island | • Residual temporal island |

**5. Medical therapy**

| **DRUGS TO TREAT GLAUCOMA** |
|---|
| 1. Beta-blockers |
| 2. Sympathomimetics |
| 3. Miotics |
| 4. Prostaglandin analogues |
| 5. Carbonic anhydrase inhibitors |
|    • Topical |
|    • Systemic |

**6. Laser trabeculo-plasty**

| **Indications** |
|---|
| ● Failed medical therapy |
| ● Primary therapy in non-compliant patients |
| **Technique** |

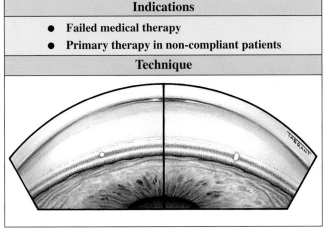

| | |
|---|---|
| • Application of 50–100 burns to junction of pigmented and non-pigmented trabeculum | • Incorrect focus with oval aiming beam |
| • Correct focus with round aiming beam | |

## 7. Trabeculec-tomy

**Indications**

1. Failed medical therapy and laser trabeculoplasty
2. Lack of suitability for trabeculoplasty
   - Poor patient co-operation
   - Inability to adequately visualize trabeculum
3. As primary therapy in advanced disease

**Technique**

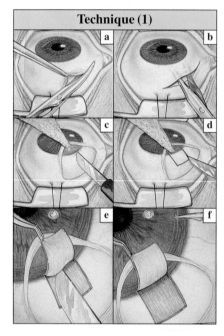

### Technique (1)

- Conjunctival incision (a)

- Conjunctival undermining (b)

- Clearing of limbus (c)

- Outline of superficial flap (d)

- Dissection of superficial flap (e)

- Paracentesis (f)

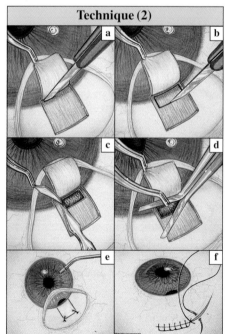

### Technique (2)

- Cutting of deep block anterior incision (a)

- Posterior incision (b)

- Excision of deep block (c)

- Peripheral iridectomy (d)

- Suturing of flap and reconstitution of anterior chamber (e)

- Suturing of conjunctiva (f)

**Filtration blebs**

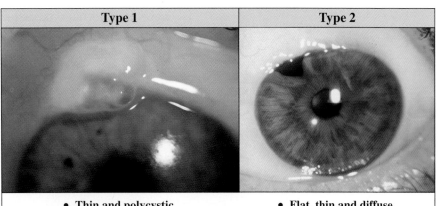

| Type 1 | Type 2 |
|---|---|
| • Thin and polycystic<br>• Good filtration | • Flat, thin and diffuse<br>• Microcysts present<br>• Good filtration |

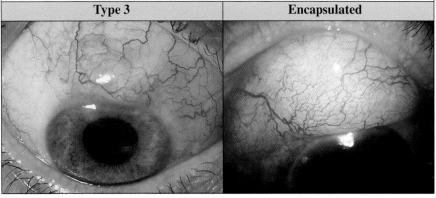

| Type 3 | Encapsulated |
|---|---|
| • Flat<br>• Engorged surface vessels<br>• No microcysts<br>• No filtration | • Localized, firm cyst<br>• Engorged surface vessels<br>• No filtration |

**Complications**

| SHALLOW ANTERIOR CHAMBER | | | |
|---|---|---|---|
| **Cause** | **IOP** | **Bleb** | **Seidel test** |
| Wound leak | Low | Poor | Positive |
| Overfiltration | Low | Good | Negative |
| Malignant glaucoma | High | Poor | Negative |

| Late bleb infection – predispositions | |
|---|---|
| • Thin-walled, cystic bleb<br>• Use of adjunctive antimetabolites<br>• Bleb trauma | |
| **Blebitis** | **Endophthalmitis** |

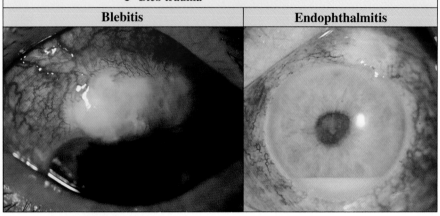

| | |
|---|---|
| • Subacute onset<br>• Milky bleb<br>• No hypopyon<br>• Good prognosis | • Acute onset<br>• Hypopyon<br>• Guarded prognosis |

# PRIMARY ANGLE-CLOSURE GLAUCOMA

1. Pathogenesis

2. Classification

3. Intermittent

4. Acute congestive

5. Postcongestive

6. Chronic

## 1. Pathogenesis

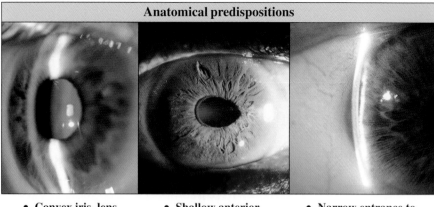

**Anatomical predispositions**

- Convex iris–lens diaphragm
- Shallow anterior chamber
- Narrow entrance to chamber angle

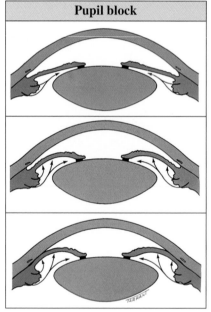

**Pupil block**

- Increase in physiological pupil block

- Dilatation of pupil renders peripheral iris more flaccid
- Increased pressure in posterior chamber causes iris bombé

- Angle obstructed by peripheral iris and rise in IOP

## 2. Classification

1. Latent – asymptomatic
   - IOP may remain normal
   - May progress to subacute, acute or chronic angle closure
2. Subacute – intermittent angle closure
   - May develop acute or chronic angle closure
3. Acute
   - Congestive – sudden total angle closure
   - Postcongestive – follows acute attack
4. Chronic – 'creeping' angle closure
   - Follows intermittent or latent angle closure
5. Absolute
   - No PL following acute attack

**3. Intermittent**

| Signs | Treatment |
|---|---|
| 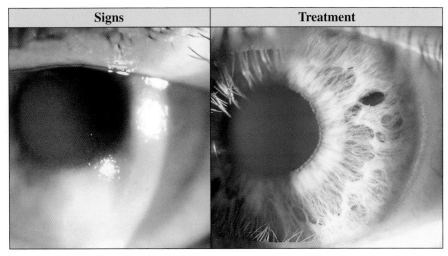 | |
| • Epithelial oedema and closed angle during attack | • Bilateral YAG laser iridotomy |

**4. Acute congestive**

| Signs |
|---|
| 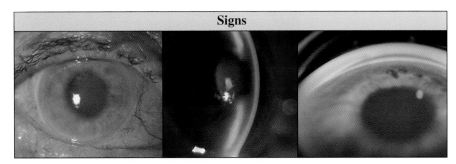 |

- Severe corneal oedema
- Dilated, unreactive, vertically oval pupil
- Ciliary injection
- Shallow anterior chamber
- Complete angle closure (Shaffer grade 0)

---

**TREATMENT**

1. Acetazolamide 500 mg i.v.
2. Hyperosmotic agents – if appropriate
   - Oral glycerol 1–1.5 g/kg of 50% solution in lemon juice
   - Intravenous mannitol 2 g/kg of 20% solution
3. Topical therapy
   - Pilocarpine 2% to both eyes
   - Beta-blockers
   - Steroids
4. YAG laser iridotomy
   - To both eyes when cornea is clear

## 5. Post-congestive

| Signs |
|---|
| 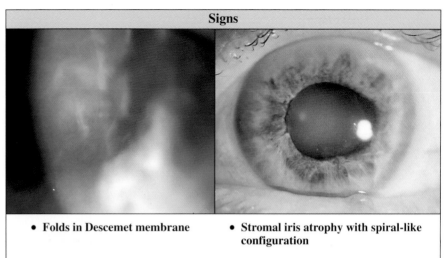 |
| • Folds in Descemet membrane      • Stromal iris atrophy with spiral-like configuration |
| 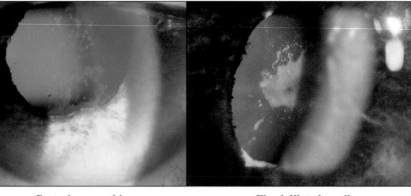 |
| • Posterior synechiae      • Fixed dilated pupil |
| • Fine pigment on iris      • Glaukomflecken |

## 6. Chronic

| Signs |
|---|
| 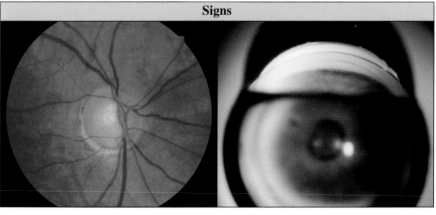 |
| • Similar to POAG with cupping and field loss      • Easily missed unless routine gonioscopy performed |
|      • Variable amount of angle closure |

# SECONDARY GLAUCOMAS

1. **Pseudoexfoliation glaucoma**

2. **Pigmentary glaucoma**

3. **Neovascular glaucoma**

4. **Inflammatory glaucomas**

5. **Phacolytic glaucoma**

6. **Post-traumatic angle recession glaucoma**

7. **Iridocorneal endothelial syndrome**

8. **Glaucoma associated with iridoschisis**

## 1. Pseudo-exfoliation glaucoma

- Secondary trabecular block open-angle glaucoma
- Affects elderly, unilateral in 60%
- Prognosis less good than in POAG

| Pseudoexfoliative material | Iris sphincter atrophy | Gonioscopy |
|---|---|---|
| 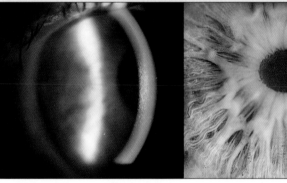 | | |
| - Central disc with peripheral band | - On retroillumination | - Trabecular hyperpigmentation – may extend anteriorly (Sampaolesi line) |

## 2. Pigmentary glaucoma

- Bilateral trabecular block open-angle glaucoma
- Typically affects young myopic males
- Increased incidence of lattice degeneration

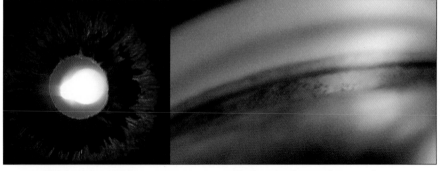

- Krukenberg spindle and very deep anterior chamber
- Fine pigment granules on anterior iris surface

- Mid-peripheral iris atrophy
- Trabecular hyperpigmentation

## 3. Neovascular glaucoma

| Causes |
| --- |
| ● Common, secondary angle-closure glaucoma without pupil block |
| ● Caused by rubeosis iridis associated with chronic, diffuse retinal ischaemia |

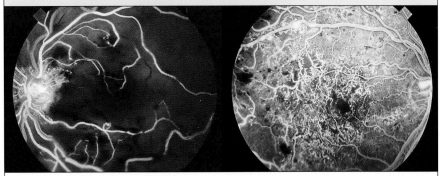

● Ischaemic central retinal vein occlusion (most common)

● Longstanding diabetes (common)

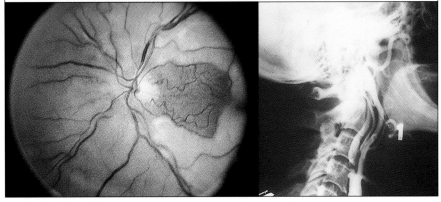

● Central retinal artery occlusion (uncommon)

● Carotid obstructive disease (uncommon)

| Signs (1) |
| --- |

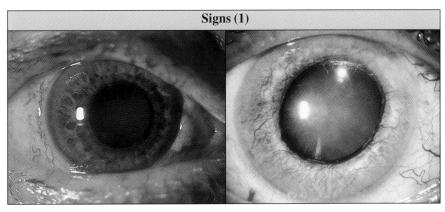

● Severely reduced visual acuity, congestion and pain

● Severe rubeosis iridis

## Signs (2)

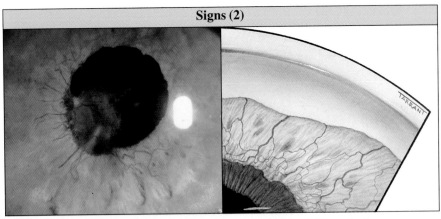

- Distortion of pupil and ectropion uveae
- Synechial angle closure

## Treatment options

- Atropine and steroids to decrease inflammation
- Beta-blockers

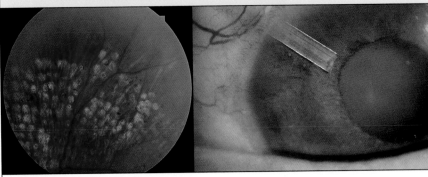

- Panretinal photocoagulation
  – in early cases
- Artificial filtering devices
  – in very advanced cases

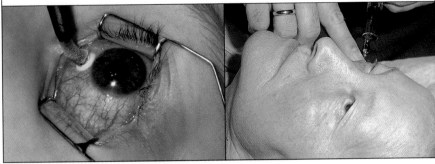

- Cyclodestructive procedures
  – to relieve pain
- Retrobulbar alcohol injection
  – to relieve pain

## 4. Inflammatory glaucomas

**Angle closure with pupil block**

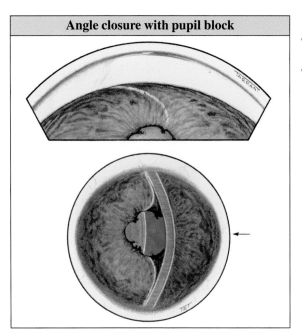

- Caused by seclusio pupillae
- Anterior chamber is shallow

**Angle closure without pupil block**

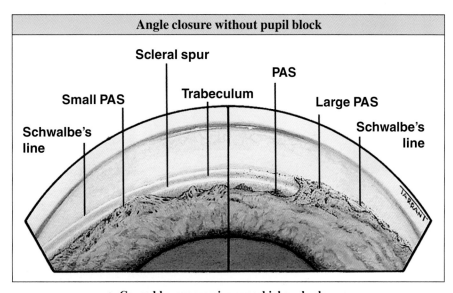

Scleral spur

PAS

Small PAS

Trabeculum

Large PAS

Schwalbe's line

Schwalbe's line

- Caused by progressive synechial angle closure
- Anterior chamber is deep

## 5. Phacolytic glaucoma

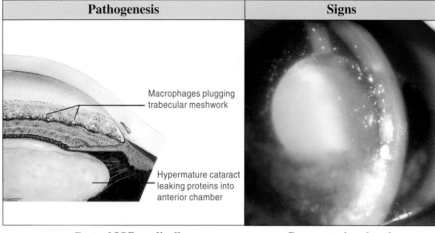

| Pathogenesis | Signs |
|---|---|
| Macrophages plugging trabecular meshwork | |
| Hypermature cataract leaking proteins into anterior chamber | |

*Treatment*

- Control IOP medically
- Remove cataract

- Deep anterior chamber
- Floating white particles

## 6. Post-traumatic angle recession glaucoma

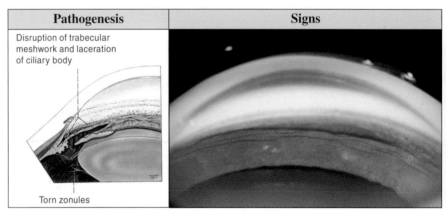

| Pathogenesis | Signs |
|---|---|
| Disruption of trabecular meshwork and laceration of ciliary body | |
| Torn zonules | |

- Blunt traumatic damage to trabecular meshwork

- Irregular widening of ciliary body band

## 7. Iridocorneal endothelial syndrome

### CLASSIFICATION

- Proliferation of abnormal corneal endothelial cells
- Typically affects young to middle-aged women
- Three syndromes with certain overlap
  1. Progressive iris atrophy
     - Iris atrophy in 100%
  2. Iris naevus (Cogan–Reese) syndrome
     - Iris atrophy in 50%
  3. Chandler syndrome
     - Iris atrophy in 40%
     - Corneal changes predominate

## Progressive iris atrophy

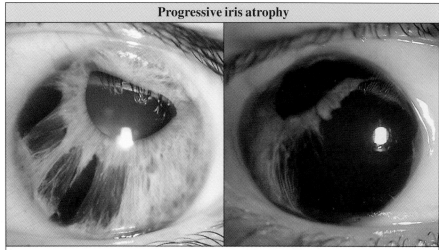

- Progressive stromal iris atrophy

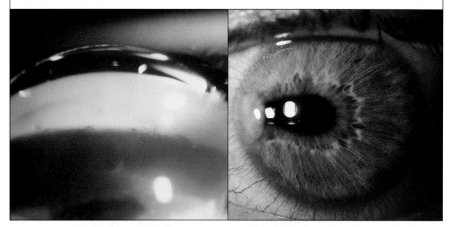

- Broad-based PAS
- Displacement of pupil towards PAS

## Iris naevus (Cogan–Reese) syndrome

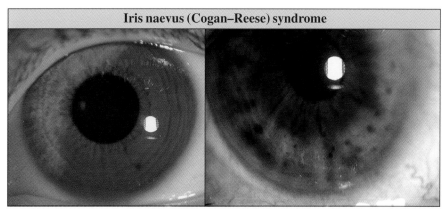

- Diffuse iris naevus
- Pedunculated iris nodules

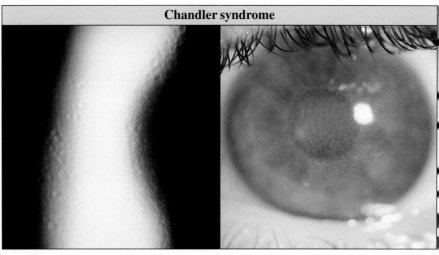

**Chandler syndrome**

- Initially 'hammered-silver' endothelial changes

- Later oedema which may cause halos

## 8. Glaucoma associated with iridoschisis

- Rare, affects elderly, often bilateral
- Underlying, angle-closure glaucoma in about 90%

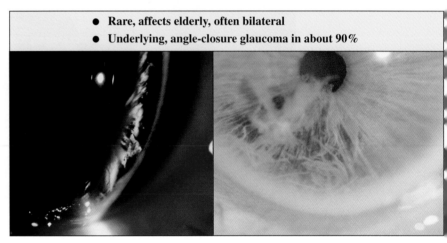

- Shallow anterior chamber

- Iridoschisis – usually inferior

# CONGENITAL GLAUCOMAS

1. **Primary**

2. **Iridocorneal dysgenesis**
   - Axenfeld–Rieger anomaly
   - Peters anomaly
   - Aniridia

3. **In phacomatoses**
   - Sturge–Weber syndrome
   - Neurofibromatosis – 1

## 1. Primary

- 1:10 000 births, 65% boys
- Most sporadic – 10% autosomal recessive
- Absence of angle recess with iris inserted directly into trabeculum

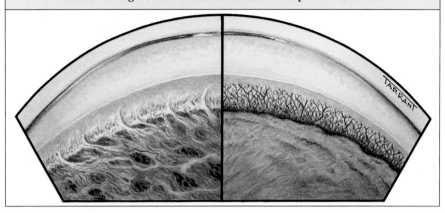

- Flat iris insertion
- Concave iris insertion

| Clinical features |
|---|

- Depend on age of onset
- Bilateral in 75% but frequently asymmetrical

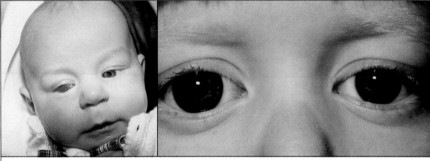

- Corneal oedema associated with lacrimation and photophobia
- Buphthalmos if IOP becomes elevated prior to age 3 years

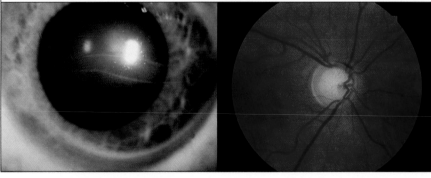

- Breaks in Descemet membrane
- Optic disc cupping

| Management | | |
|---|---|---|
| **Measurement of IOP and corneal diameters** | **Goniotomy** | **Trabeculotomy** |

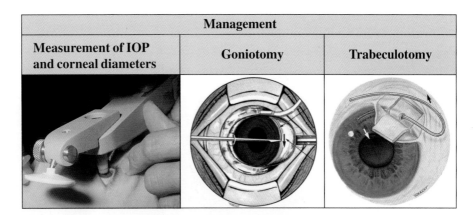

## 2. Iridocorneal dysgenesis

**Axenfeld–Rieger anomaly**

| Axenfeld anomaly |
|---|
| ● Bilateral but asymmetrical |
| ● Glaucoma is uncommon |

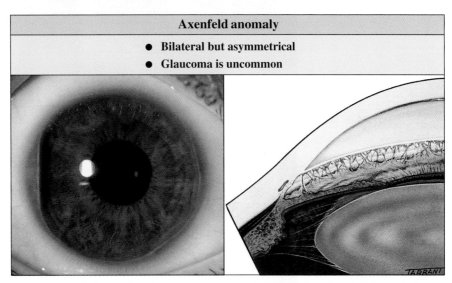

● Posterior embryotoxon

● Attached strands of iris to posterior embryotoxon

## Rieger anomaly

- Autosomal dominant
- Bilateral but asymmetrical
- Glaucoma in 50%

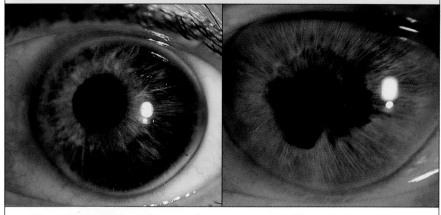

- Stromal hypoplasia and corectopia
- Ectropion uveae

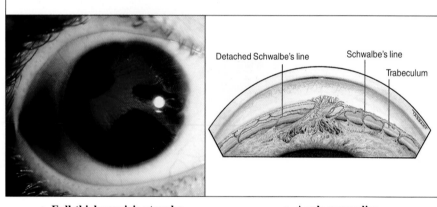

- Full-thickness iris atrophy
- Angle anomalies

## Rieger syndrome

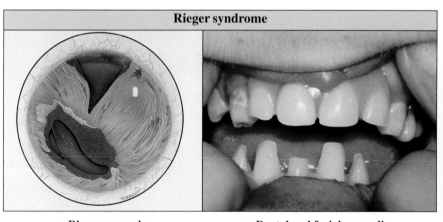

- Rieger anomaly
- Dental and facial anomalies

**Peters anomaly**

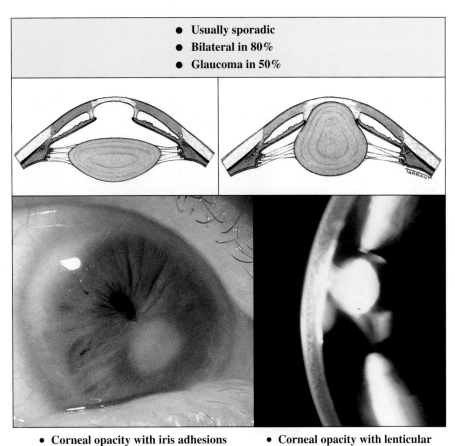

- Usually sporadic
- Bilateral in 80%
- Glaucoma in 50%

- Corneal opacity with iris adhesions
- Corneal opacity with lenticular adhesions

**Aniridia**

| SYSTEMIC IMPLICATIONS |
|---|
| **AN-1 – 85%** |
| • Autosomal dominant |
| • Isolated |
| **AN-2 (Miller syndrome) – 13%** |
| • Deletion of short arm of chromosome 11 |
| • Wilm tumour, genitourinary anomalies and mental handicap |
| **AN-3 (Gillespie syndrome) – 2%** |
| • Autosomal recessive |
| • Mental handicap and cerebellar ataxia |

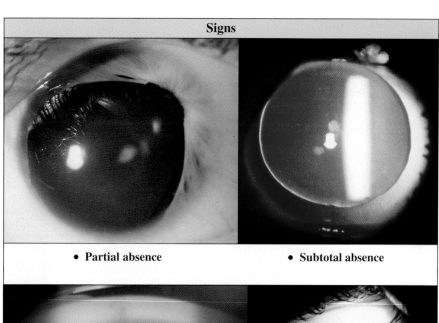

| Signs | |
|---|---|
| • Partial absence | • Subtotal absence |
| • Synechial angle-closure glaucoma in 75% | • Occasional cataract and lens subluxation |

## 3. In phaco-matoses

**Sturge–Weber syndrome**

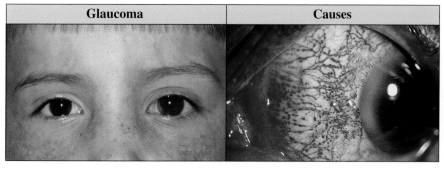

| Glaucoma | Causes |
|---|---|
| • Glaucoma in 30%<br>• Ipsilateral to facial haemangioma<br>• Buphthalmos in 60% | • Caused by raised episcleral venous pressure associated with episcleral haemangioma<br>• Angle anomaly may also be responsible |

**Neurofibro-matosis – 1**

| Glaucoma | Causes |
|---|---|
| 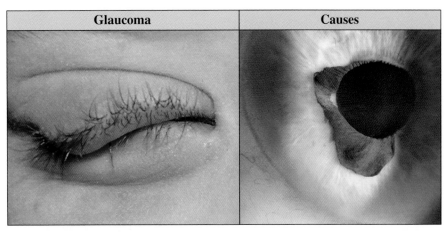 | |

- Glaucoma is ipsilateral to neurofibroma of upper eyelid in 50% of cases

- Caused by angle anomaly with or without ectropion uveae
- Angle neurofibroma may also be responsible

# IMPORTANT SYSTEMIC ASSOCIATIONS OF UVEITIS

1. **Spondylarthropathies**

2. **Juvenile idiopathic arthritis**

3. **Sarcoidosis**
   - Systemic features
   - Ocular features

4. **Behçet disease**
   - Systemic features
   - Ocular features

5. **Vogt–Koyanagi–Harada syndrome**

6. **Inflammatory bowel disease**
   - Ulcerative colitis
   - Crohn disease

7. **Tubulointerstitial nephritis and uveitis**

# 1. Spondylar-thropathies

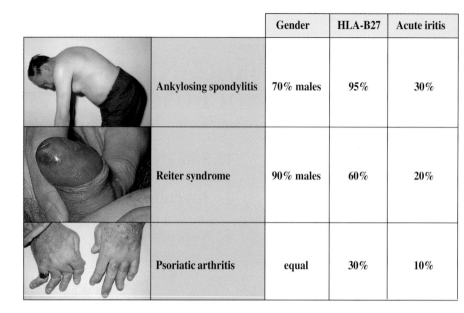

| | | Gender | HLA-B27 | Acute iritis |
|---|---|---|---|---|
| | Ankylosing spondylitis | 70% males | 95% | 30% |
| | Reiter syndrome | 90% males | 60% | 20% |
| | Psoriatic arthritis | equal | 30% | 10% |

| | Sacroiliitis | | Peripheral arthritis | Bowel inflammation |
|---|---|---|---|---|
| • Ankylosing spondylitis | | 100% | 20% | Common |
| • Reiter syndrome | | 60% | 100% | Uncommon |
| • Psoriatic arthritis | | 30% | 100% | Occasional |

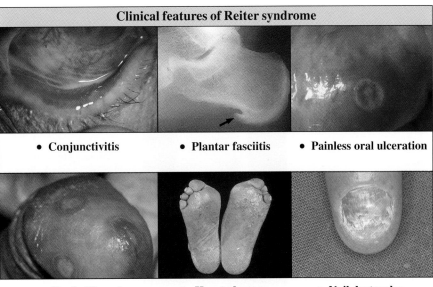

**Clinical features of Reiter syndrome**

- Conjunctivitis
- Plantar fasciitis
- Painless oral ulceration
- Urethritis and circinate balanitis
- Keratoderma blenorrhagica
- Nail dystrophy

## 2. Juvenile idiopathic arthritis

| Classification | | |
|---|---|---|
| Pauciarticular onset (60%) | Polyarticular onset (20%) | Systemic onset (20%) |

| | Pauciarticular onset (60%) | Polyarticular onset (20%) | Systemic onset (20%) |
|---|---|---|---|
| Joints (no.) | < 5 | > 4 | Variable |
| JCI onset | < 6 years | Variable | Variable |
| Systemic features | Absent | Mild or absent | Severe |
| Positive ANA | 75% | 40% | 10% |
| Iridocyclitis | 20% | 5% | Absent |

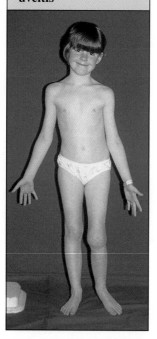

- Girls

- Early onset

- Pauciarticular onset

- ANA

- HLA-DR5

## Complications of uveitis

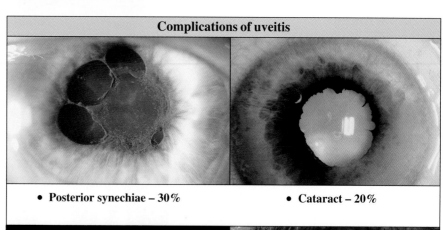

- Posterior synechiae – 30%

- Cataract – 20%

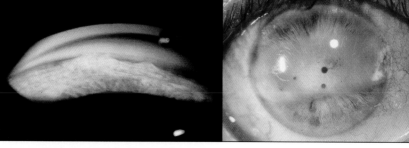

- Glaucoma due to PAS – 15%

- Band keratopathy – 10%

## 3. Sarcoidosis

**Systemic features**

| SYSTEMIC FEATURES |
|---|
| 1. Idiopathic, multisystem non-caseating granuloma |
| 2. More common in blacks than whites |
| 3. Presentation |
|    • Acute – third decade |
|    • Insidious – fifth decade |
| 4. Organ involvement |
|    • Lungs – 95% |
|    • Thoracic lymph nodes – 50% |
|    • Skin – 30% |
|    • Eyes – 30% |

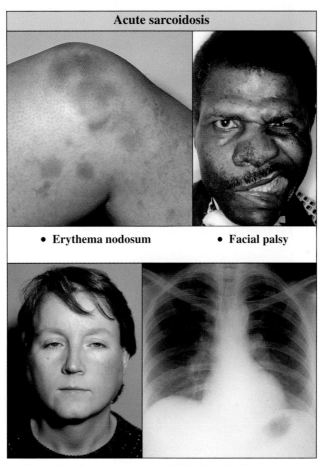

**Acute sarcoidosis**

- Erythema nodosum     • Facial palsy

- Parotid enlargement     • Hilar lymphadenopathy

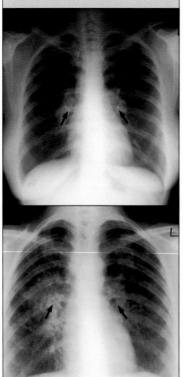

**Staging of sarcoid lung lesions**

*Stage 1*
- Hilar
- Lymphadenopathy

*Stage 2*
- Hilar
- Lymphadenopathy and parenchymal infiltrates

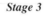

*Stage 3*
- Parenchymal
- Infiltrates alone

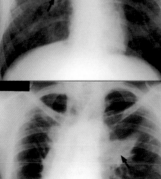

*Stage 4*
- Fibrosis and
- Bronchiectasis

| Sarcoid skin lesions | |
| --- | --- |
| **Granulomata** | **Lupus pernio** |

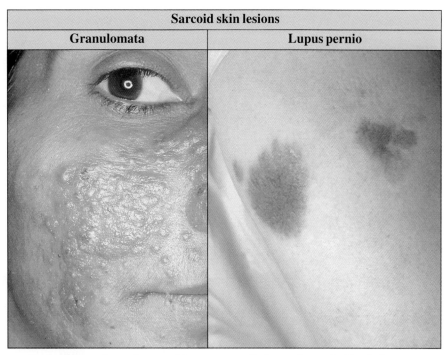

| | |
| --- | --- |
| • On face, buttocks and extremities | • Indurated, purple-blue lesions |

**Ocular features**

| Anterior segment lesions |
| --- |

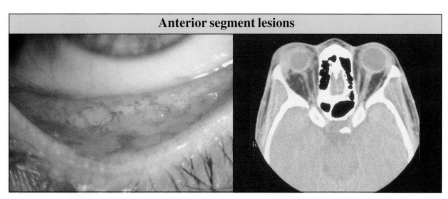

| | |
| --- | --- |
| • Conjunctival granuloma | • Lacrimal gland involvement and dry eyes |

| Iridocyclitis | |
|---|---|
| **Acute non-granulomatous** | **Chronic granulomatous** |

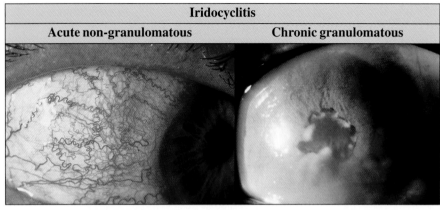

| | |
|---|---|
| • In young patients with acute sarcoid | • In older patients with chronic sarcoid |

**Posterior segment lesions**

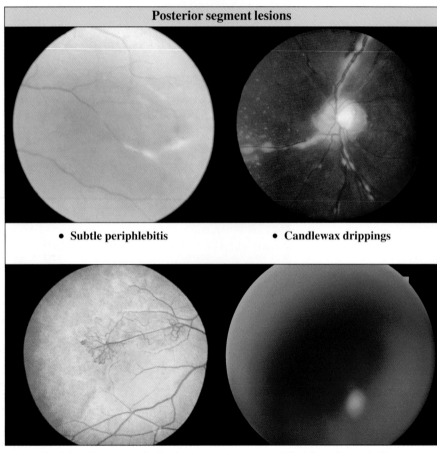

| | |
|---|---|
| • Subtle periphlebitis | • Candlewax drippings |
| • Peripheral neovascularization | • Vitritis and snowballs |

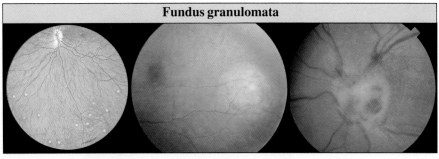

**Fundus granulomata**

- Retinal and preretinal
- Choroidal
- Optic nerve head

## 4. Behçet disease

**Systemic features**

**BEHÇET DISEASE**

1. Idiopathic multisystem disease
2. Presentation – third to fourth decade
3. Most prevalent in Mediterranean region and Japan
4. Associated with HLA-B5 in Turkey and Japan
5. Major diagnostic criteria
   - Oral aphthous ulceration (100%)
   - Genital ulceration (90%)
   - Skin lesions (80%)
   - Uveitis (70%)

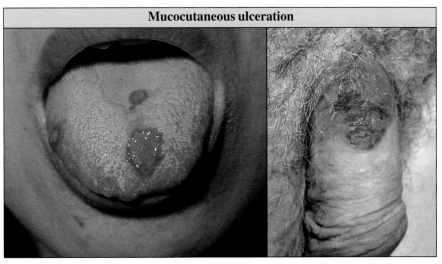

**Mucocutaneous ulceration**

- Oral aphthous ulceration – painful, recurrent
- Genital ulceration

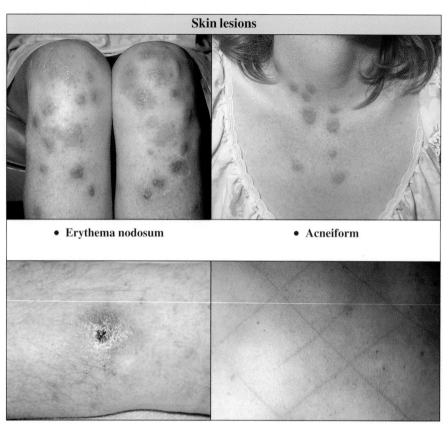

**Skin lesions**

- Erythema nodosum

- Acneiform

- Pustule after scratching skin
  (pathergy test)

- Lines after stroking skin
  (dermatographism)

**Vascular lesions**

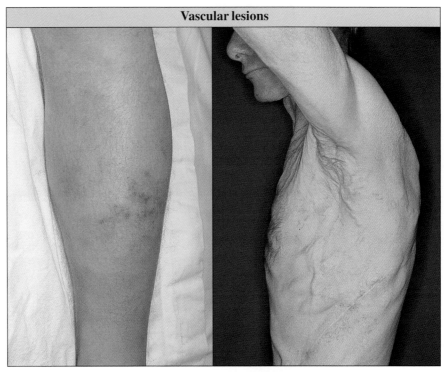

- Migratory thrombophlebitis of extremities
- Obliterative thrombophlebitis of major internal veins

**Ocular features**

**Uveitis (1)**

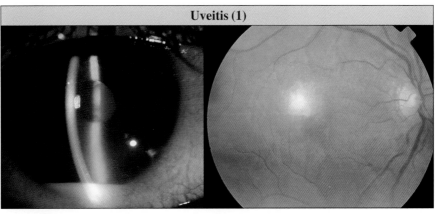

- Acute iritis
- Retinitis

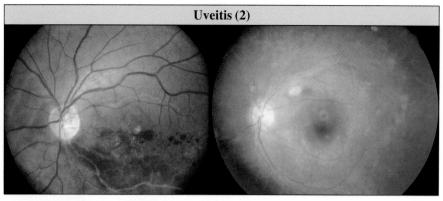

## Uveitis (2)

- Occlusive periphlebitis
- Diffuse leakage

5. Vogt–
Koyanagi–
Harada
syndrome

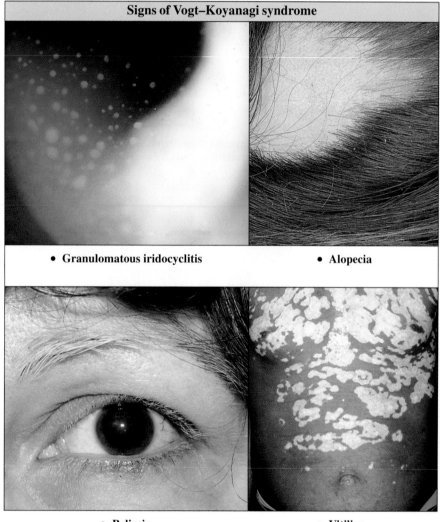

## Signs of Vogt–Koyanagi syndrome

- Granulomatous iridocyclitis
- Alopecia
- Poliosis
- Vitiligo

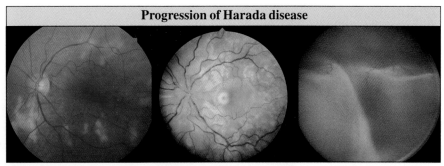

**Progression of Harada disease**

- Multifocal choroiditis
- Multifocal sensory retinal detachments
- Exudative retinal detachment

## 6. Inflammatory bowel disease

**Ulcerative colitis**

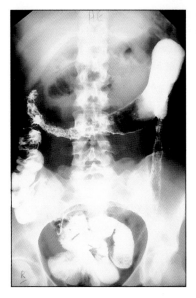

- Large bowel ulceration
- Acute iritis – uncommon

**Crohn disease**

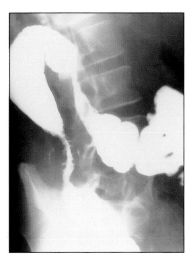

- Stricture and 'rose thorn' ulceration
- Acute iritis – uncommon

## 7. Tubulointer-stitial nephritis and uveitis

| Renal histology | Urine |
|---|---|
| 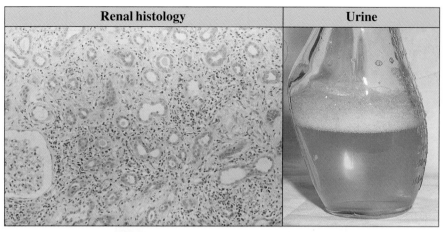 | |

- Most frequently affects women and children
- Hypersensitivity reaction to drugs
- Bilateral, recurrent anterior uveitis

- Proteinuria and renal failure
- Good response to systemic steroids

# UVEAL INFECTIONS AND INFESTATIONS

1. **Viruses**
   - Herpes zoster ophthalmicus
   - Acute retinal necrosis
   - Cytomegalovirus

2. **Acquired immune deficiency syndrome**
   - Systemic features
   - Ocular features

3. **Spirochaetes**
   - Syphilis
   - Lyme disease

4. **Mycobacteria**
   - Tuberculosis
   - Leprosy

5. **Protozoa and worms**
   - Toxoplasmosis
   - Ocular toxocariasis

6. **Fungi**
   - Presumed ocular histoplasmosis syndrome
   - Candidiasis

## 1. Viruses

**Herpes zoster ophthalmicus**

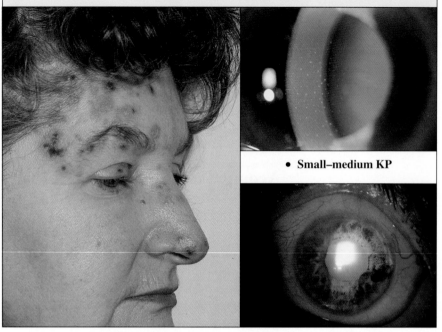

- Iritis in 40% of cases
- Within 3 weeks of onset of rash

- Small–medium KP

- Particularly if external nasal branch involved – Hutchinson sign
- Iris atrophy – 20%

**Acute retinal necrosis**

- Affects healthy individuals (bilateral in 30–50%)
- Herpes simplex in young patients
- Herpes zoster in older patients

### Signs

- Peripheral vasculitis
- Deep, multifocal, yellow, necrotic infiltrates

- Vitritis and anterior uveitis

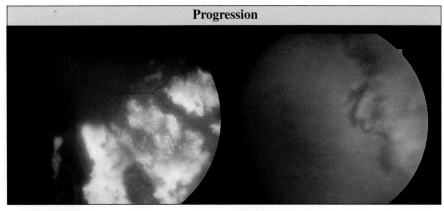

**Progression**

- Confluence but sparing of posterior pole until late
- Residual RPE atrophy after 4–12 weeks

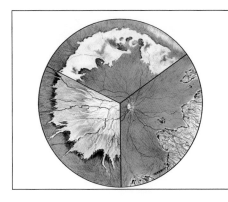

*Treatment options*
- Systemic aciclovir, steroids, aspirin
- Laser photocoagulation to limit progression

*Complications*
- Retinal detachment
- Ischaemic optic neuropathy

## 2. Acquired immune deficiency syndrome (AIDS)

### Systemic features

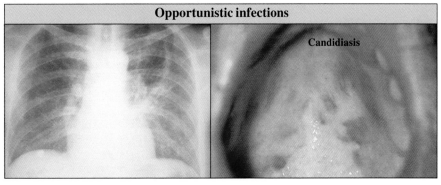

Candidiasis

- *Pneumocystis carinii* pneumonia
- Toxoplasmosis
- Atypical mycobacterium
- Cytomegalovirus
- Cryptococcus

| Neoplasms |
| --- |

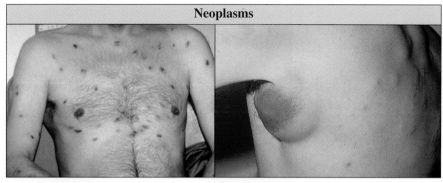

- Kaposi sarcoma       • Lymphoma

**Ocular features**

| Anterior features |
| --- |

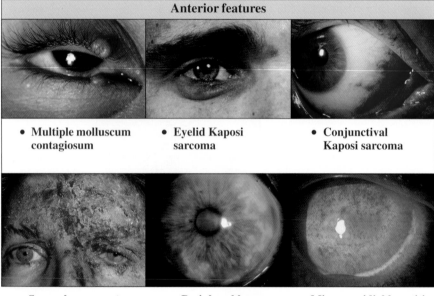

- Multiple molluscum contagiosum
- Eyelid Kaposi sarcoma
- Conjunctival Kaposi sarcoma

- Severe herpes zoster ophthalmicus
- Peripheral herpes simplex keratitis
- Microsporidial keratitis

## HIV retinal microangiopathy

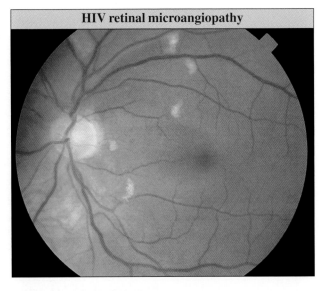

- In 66% of AIDS
- In 40% of AIDS-related complex
- In 1% of asymptomatic HIV infection
- Transient cotton-wool spots
- Occasionally haemorrhages

## Indolent CMV retinitis

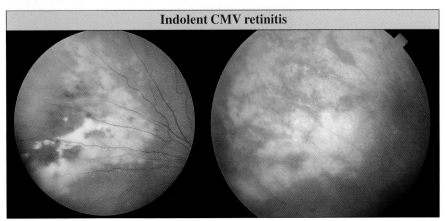

- Frequently starts in periphery
- Granular opacification

- Slow progression
- No vasculitis
- Mild vitritis

## Fulminating CMV retinitis

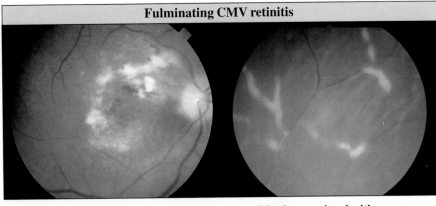

- Dense, white, confluent opacification
- Frequently along vascular arcades
- Associated haemorrhages
- May be associated with venous sheathing
- Mild vitritis

## Progression of CMV retinitis

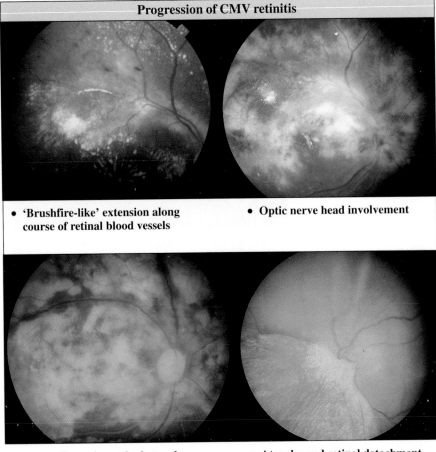

- 'Brushfire-like' extension along course of retinal blood vessels
- Optic nerve head involvement
- Extensive retinal atrophy
- Atrophy and retinal detachment

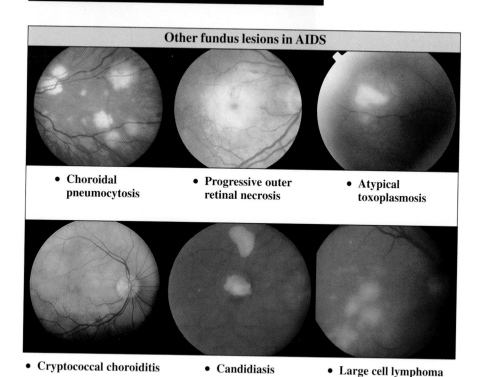

## Treatment of CMV retinitis

*Ganciclovir*

- Systemic – initially i.v. then oral
- Intravitreal – injections or slow-release devices

*Foscarnet i.v.*

*Cidofovir i.v.*

*Signs of regression*

- Fewer haemorrhages
- Less opacification
- Diffuse atrophic and pigmentary changes

## Other fundus lesions in AIDS

- Choroidal pneumocytosis
- Progressive outer retinal necrosis
- Atypical toxoplasmosis
- Cryptococcal choroiditis
- Candidiasis
- Large cell lymphoma

## 3. Spirochaetes

### Syphilis

- Infection with spirochaete *Treponema pallidum*
- Uveitis may occur during secondary and tertiary stages
- Uncommon, bilateral in 50%

### Iridocyclitis

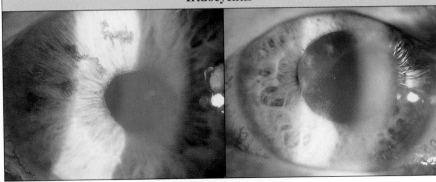

- Initially may be associated with dilated vessels (roseolae)

- Becomes chronic unless treated

### Posterior uveitis

| Unifocal chorioretinitis | Multifocal chorioretinitis |
|---|---|

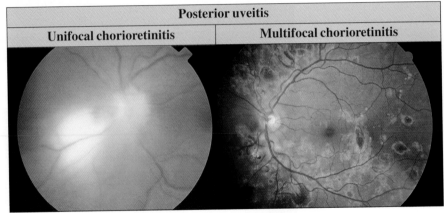

- May be bilateral
- Frequently juxtapapillary or central

- May be bilateral
- Residual choroidal atrophy and RPE changes

| Acute neuroretinitis | Inactive neuroretinitis |
|---|---|

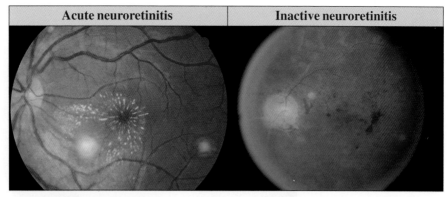

- Usually unilateral
- Disc oedema, macular star and cotton-wool spots

- Optic atrophy, vascular non-perfusion and RPE changes

**Lyme disease**

- Infection with *Borrelia burgdorferi*
- Transmitted through bite of tick *Ixodes* sp.
- Early and late manifestations

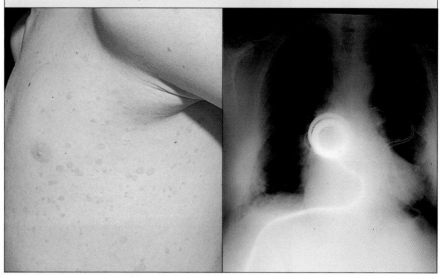

- Skin rash (erythema migrans)

- Cardiac conduction defects

| CNS lesions | Monoarthritis |
|---|---|

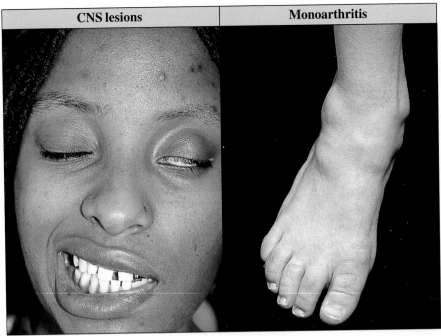

| Ocular features |
|---|

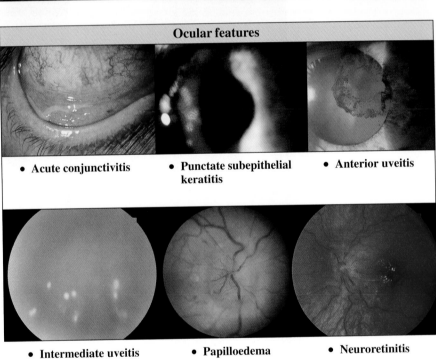

- Acute conjunctivitis
- Punctate subepithelial keratitis
- Anterior uveitis

- Intermediate uveitis
- Papilloedema
- Neuroretinitis

## 4. Mycobacteria

**Tuberculosis**

- Infection with human (*Mycobacterium tuberculosis*) or bovine (*M. bovis*)
- Uveitis is uncommon and occurs during post-primary stage

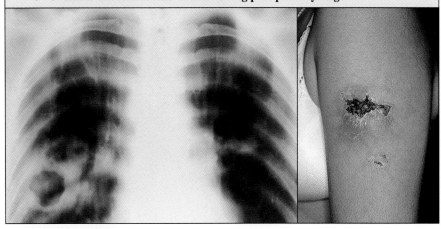

- Lung cavitation
- Negative chest X-ray does not exclude TB

- Positive skin test
- Useful in diagnosis of extrathoracic TB

### Chronic granulomatous iridocyclitis

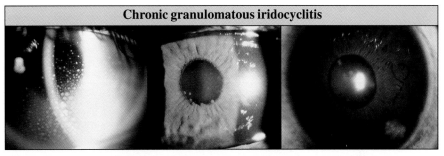

- Mutton fat KP
- Koeppe nodules
- Busacca nodules

### Posterior uveitis

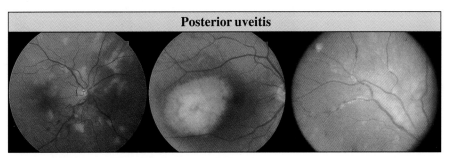

- Choroiditis – unifocal or multifocal
- Large solitary choroidal granuloma
- Retinal periphlebitis

**Leprosy**

- Infection with *M. leprae*
- Two types of leprosy – lepromatous and tuberculoid
- Affinity for skin, peripheral nerves and eye

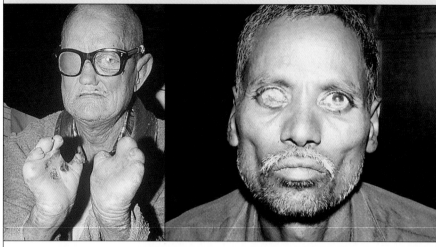

- Neurological involvement
- Severe corneal scarring

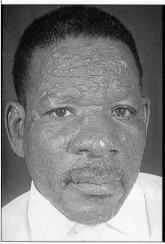
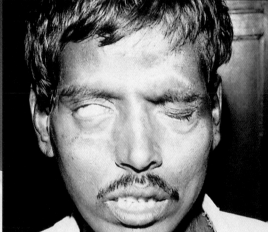

- Madarosis and skin involvement
- Lagophthalmos

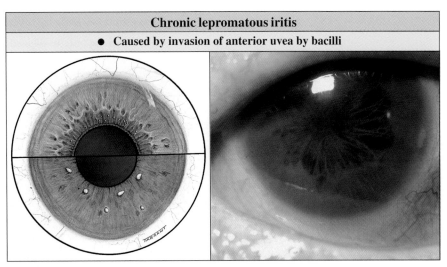

**Chronic lepromatous iritis**

● Caused by invasion of anterior uvea by bacilli

● Initially small, peripupillary, glistening 'iris pearls'

● Pearls enlarge and drop into anterior chamber

● Eventual iris atrophy, miosis and cataract

## 5. Protozoa and worms

### Toxoplasmosis

**Life cycle**

● Intracellular protozoan *Toxoplasma gondii*

● Cat is definitive host

● Other animals and humans are intermediate hosts

Definitive Host

Intermediate Hosts

Direct    Indirect

Oocyst in soil

Tissue cyst

Congenital Toxoplasmosis

## Congenital systemic involvement

- Severity of involvement of fetus depends on duration of gestation at time of maternal infestation

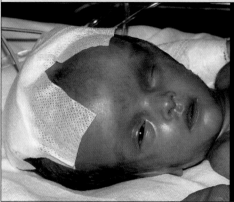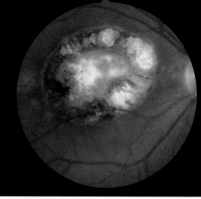

- Infestation during late pregnancy may cause hydrocephalus
- Chorioretinal scarring at macula which may be bilateral

## Toxoplasma retinitis

- Recurrence of healed congenital lesion
- Usually between ages 10 – 35 years

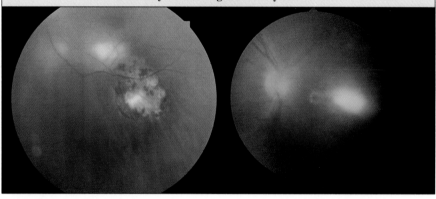

- Unifocal retinitis adjacent to old scar – heals within 1–4 months
- Vitritis may be severe – 'headlight in fog'

| Treatment of toxoplasma retinitis |
| :---: |
| **Indications** |

- Lesions at posterior pole, near optic disc or major blood vessel
- Very severe vitritis
- AIDS patients irrespective of location or severity

*Drugs*

1. Systemic steroids
2. Clindamycin
3. Sulphonamides
4. Pyrimethamide
5. Co-trimoxazole
6. Azithromycin
7. Atovaquone

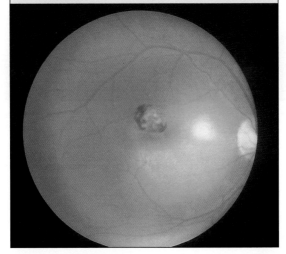

**Ocular toxocariasis**

| ● Always unilateral | |
| :---: | :---: |
| **Chronic endophthalmitis** | **Posterior pole granuloma** |

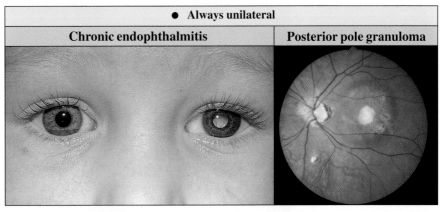

- Presents between 2 and 9 years with leukocoria or strabismus
- Presents between 6 and 14 years with visual loss

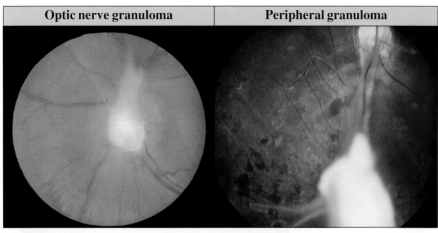

| Optic nerve granuloma | Peripheral granuloma |
|---|---|
| • Presents between 6 and 14 years with visual loss | • Presents during adolescence or adult life with visual loss |

## 6. Fungi

**Presumed ocular histoplasmosis syndrome**

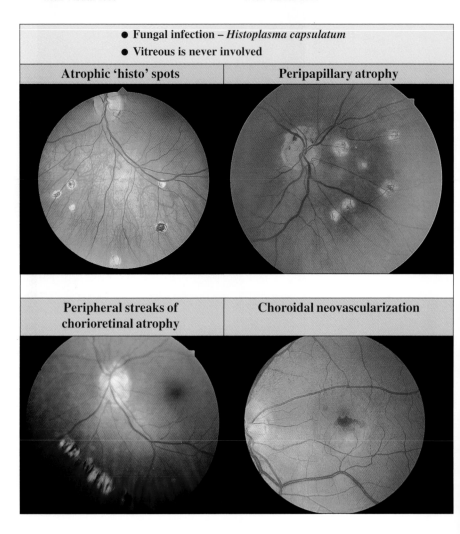

- Fungal infection – *Histoplasma capsulatum*
- Vitreous is never involved

| Atrophic 'histo' spots | Peripapillary atrophy |
|---|---|

| Peripheral streaks of chorioretinal atrophy | Choroidal neovascularization |
|---|---|

**Candidiasis**

- Infection with yeast-like fungus – *Candida albicans*

**Risk groups**

- Drug addicts or compromised host
- Patients with long-term indwelling catheters

**Progression**

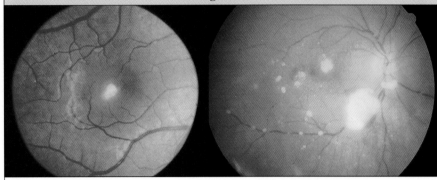

- Unifocal choroiditis
- Multifocal retinitis and vitreous 'cotton-ball' colonies

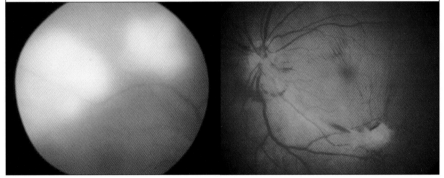

- Endophthalmitis
- Vitreoretinal traction

# IDIOPATHIC SPECIFIC UVEITIS SYNDROMES

1. **Fuchs uveitis syndrome**

2. **Intermediate uveitis**

3. **Juvenile chronic iridocyclitis**

4. **Acute anterior uveitis in young adults**

5. **Sympathetic ophthalmitis**

## 1. Fuchs uveitis syndrome

| Signs |
|---|
| • Unilateral, chronic anterior uveitis<br>• Resistant to therapy |

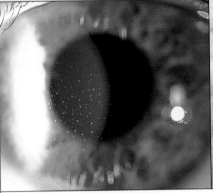

| • KP – small and scattered throughout endothelium<br>• Feathery fibrin filaments | • No posterior synechiae<br>• Diffuse iris stromal atrophy<br>• Occasionally iris nodules |
|---|---|

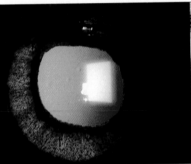 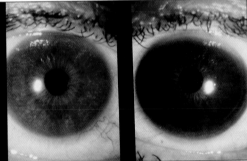

| • Iris retroillumination | • Heterochromia iridis – affected eye is usually hypochromic |
|---|---|

| Complications | | |
|---|---|---|
| Cataract | Angle new vessels | Glaucoma |

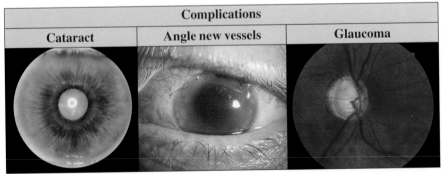

| • Very common and frequently presenting feature | • May bleed during surgery | • Uncommon but control may be difficult |
|---|---|---|

## 2. Intermediate uveitis

| Signs |
| --- |
| ● Typically affects children and young adults |
| ● Insidious and chronic |
| ● Frequently bilateral but asymmetrical |
| ● Usually presents with floaters |

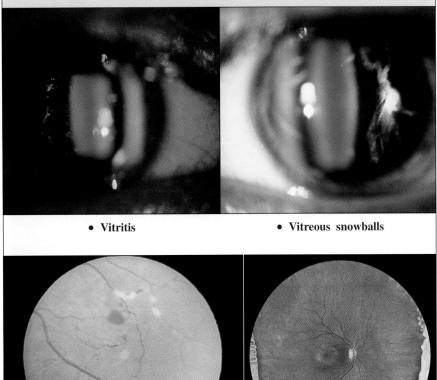

● Vitritis    ● Vitreous snowballs

● Mild peripheral periphlebitis    ● Snowbanking in pars planitis

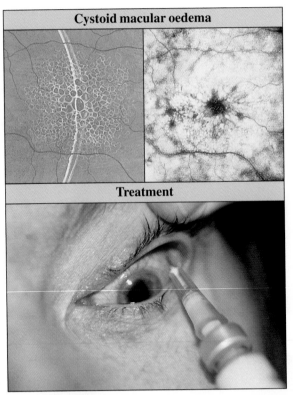

**Cystoid macular oedema**

**Treatment**

- Posterior sub-Tenon steroids if poor VA

**3. Juvenile chronic iridocyclitis**

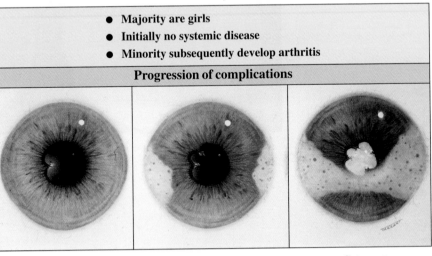

- Majority are girls
- Initially no systemic disease
- Minority subsequently develop arthritis

**Progression of complications**

- Posterior synechiae     • Band keratopathy     • Cataract

## 4. Acute anterior uveitis in young adults

- Majority are men
- 45% are positive for HLA-B27
- Initially no systemic disease
- Minority subsequently develop ankylosing spondylitis

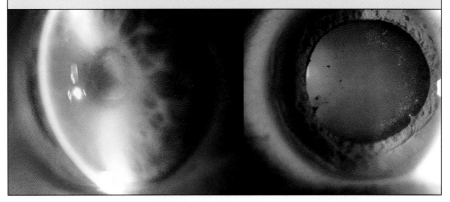

- Fibrinous exudate
- Residual pigment on lens

## 5. Sympathetic ophthalmitis

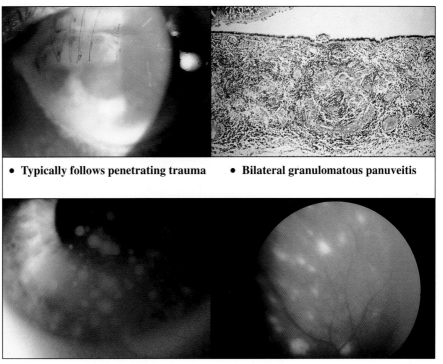

- Typically follows penetrating trauma
- Bilateral granulomatous panuveitis

- Granulomatous anterior uveitis
- Multifocal choroiditis

# IDIOPATHIC INFLAMMATORY WHITE DOT SYNDROMES

1. Multiple evanescent white dot syndrome

2. Acute posterior multifocal placoid pigment epitheliopathy

3. Punctate inner choroidopathy (PIC)

4. Birdshot retinochoroidopathy

5. Multifocal choroiditis with panuveitis

6. Serpiginous choroidopathy

## 1. Multiple evanescent white dot syndrome

- Young adults (F > M)
- Unilateral
- Small, subtle, deep grey-white dots
- Orange macular granularity
- Mild vitritis

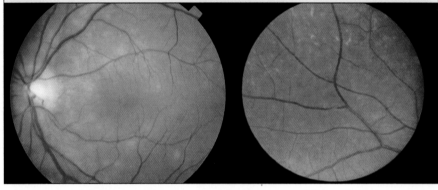

- Posterior pole
- Mid-periphery

### Fluorescein angiogram

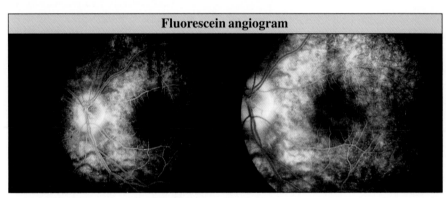

- Many hyperfluorescent spots at posterior pole
- Increase in hyperfluorescence and late leakage from disc

- Treatment – nil
- Course – 6 weeks
- Complications – nil
- Prognosis – excellent

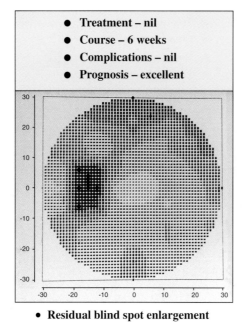

- **Residual blind spot enlargement**

## 2. Acute posterior multifocal placoid pigment epitheliopathy

- Young adults (F = M)
- Associated with HLA-B7 and DR2
- Bilateral and symmetrical

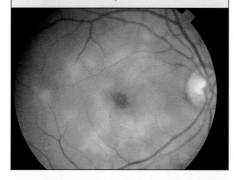

- Large, deep, grey-white, placoid lesions
- Mainly at posterior pole
- Mild vitritis

### Fluorescein angiogram

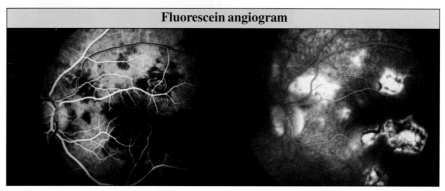

- **Early dense hypofluorescence**
- **Late staining**

- Treatment – nil
- Course – 4 weeks
- Complications – nil
- Prognosis – good

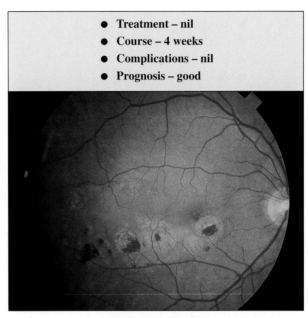

- Residual RPE changes

## 3. Punctate inner choroidopathy (PIC)

- Young, myopic females
- Eventually bilateral but asymmetrical

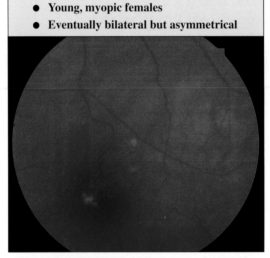

- Deep, small, indistinct yellow spots at posterior pole
- All same age
- No vitritis

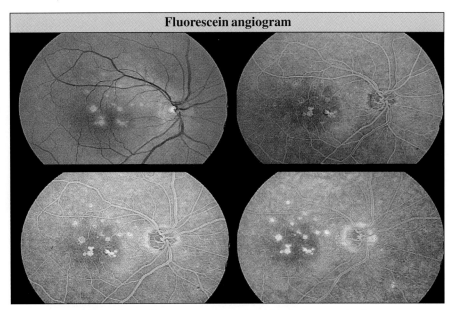

- Focal hyperfluorescent spots which do not increase in size

- Treatment – not beneficial
- Course – several weeks
- Complications – occasional (CNV)
- Prognosis – guarded

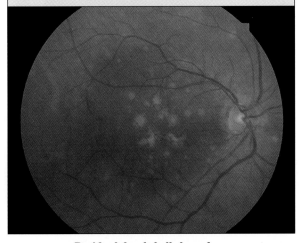

- Residual dumb-bell shaped scars

### Fluorescein angiogram of CNV in PIC

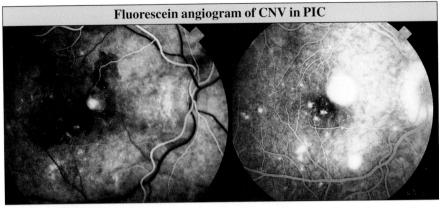

- Early hyperfluorescence
- Progressive leakage

## 4. Birdshot retinochoroidopathy

- Middle-age (F > M)
- HLA–A29

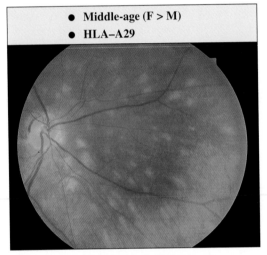

- Deep, oval, creamy, indistinct spots
- Radiate from disc towards equator
- Moderate vitritis

| Signs | Fluorescein angiogram |
|---|---|

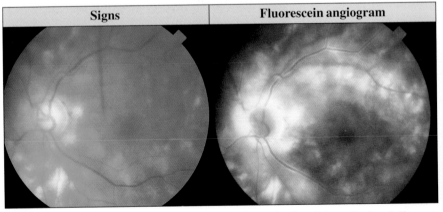

- Extensive late intraretinal and disc leakage

- Treatment – steroids and immunosuppressive agents
- Course – chronic-remittent
- Complications – CMO
- Prognosis – guarded

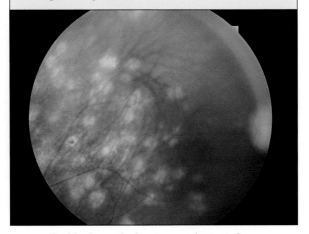

- Residual punched-out, non-pigmented scars

## 5. Multifocal choroiditis with panuveitis

- Adults (20–50 years) (F > M)
- Bilateral but asymmetrical

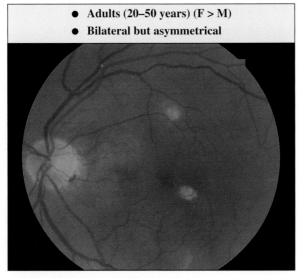

- Deep, discrete, grey-yellow spots
- Mixed fresh and old
- Mid-periphery and fewer at posterior pole
- Moderate to severe panuveitis

- Treatment – steroids
- Course – chronic-remittent
- Complications – CMO and occasional subretinal fibrosis
- Prognosis – guarded

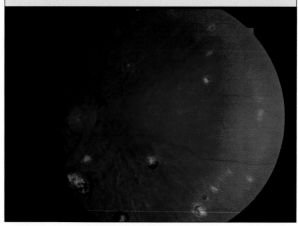

- Residual pigmented scars

## 6. Serpiginous choroidopathy

- Middle-age (F = M)
- Eventually bilateral but asymmetrical

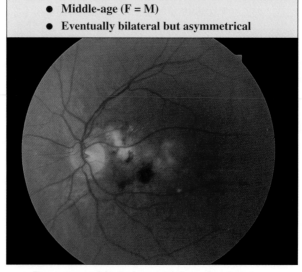

- Deep, grey-white lesions with hazy borders
- Initially peripapillary and at posterior pole then outward spread
- Mild vitritis

- **Treatment** – steroids and immunosuppressive agents
- **Course** – chronic-remittent
- **Complications** – macular scarring
- **Prognosis** – poor

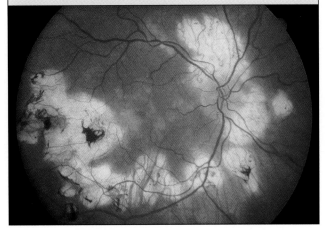

- **Residual scalloped, punched-out areas**

# UVEAL TUMOURS

1. **Iris melanoma**

2. **Iris naevus**

3. **Ciliary body melanoma**

4. **Choroidal melanoma**

5. **Choroidal naevus**

6. **Choroidal haemangioma**
   - **Circumscribed**
   - **Diffuse**

7. **Choroidal metastatic carcinoma**

8. **Choroidal osseous choristoma**

9. **Melanocytoma**

# 1. Iris melanoma

- Very rare – 8% of uveal melanomas
- Presentation – fifth to sixth decades
- Very slow growth
- Low malignancy
- Excellent prognosis

## Signs

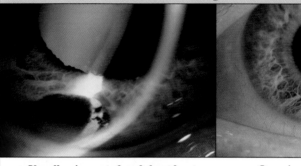

- Usually pigmented nodule at least 3 mm in diameter
- Invariably in inferior half of iris

- Occasionally non-pigmented
- Surface vascularization

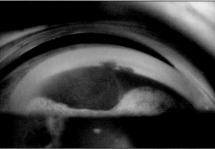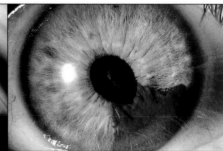

- Angle involvement may cause glaucoma

- Pupillary distortion, ectropion uveae and cataract

## Differential diagnosis (1)

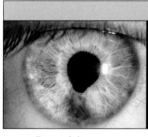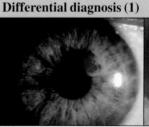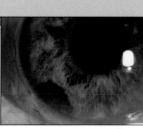

- Large iris naevus distorting pupil

- Leiomyoma

- Adenoma of pigment epithelium

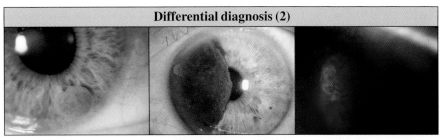

**Differential diagnosis (2)**

- Primary iris cyst
- Ciliary body melanoma eroding iris root
- Metastasis to iris

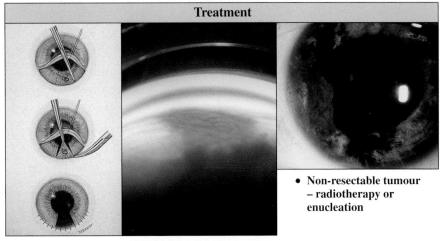

**Treatment**

- Small tumour
  – broad iridectomy
- Angle invasion by tumour
  – iridocyclectomy
- Non-resectable tumour
  – radiotherapy or enucleation

## 2. Iris naevus

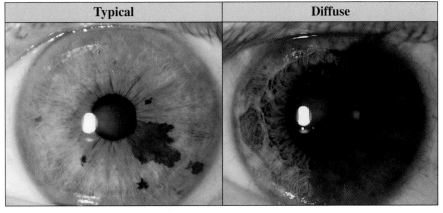

**Typical**

- Pigmented, flat or slightly elevated
- Diameter usually less than 3 mm
- Occasionally mild distortion of pupil and ectropion uvea

**Diffuse**

- Obscures iris crypts
- May cause ipsilateral hyperchromic heterochromia
- May be associated with Cogan–Reese syndrome

## 3. Ciliary body melanoma

- Rare – 12% of uveal melanomas
- Presentation – sixth decade
- May be discovered by chance
- Prognosis – guarded

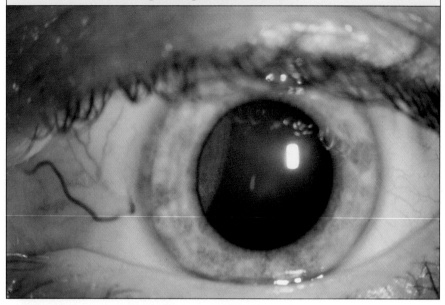

### Signs (1)

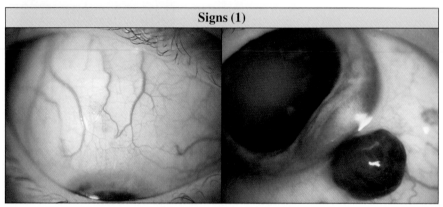

- Sentinel vessels
- Extraocular extension

## Signs (2)

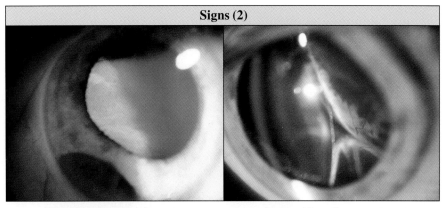

- Erosion through iris root
- Lens subluxation or cataract
- Retinal detachment

## TREATMENT OPTIONS OF CILIARY BODY MELANOMA

1. **Iridocyclectomy**
   – small or medium tumours
2. **Enucleation**
   – large tumours
3. **Radiotherapy**
   – selected cases

4. Choroidal melanoma

- Most common primary intraocular tumour in adults
- Most common uveal melanoma – 80% of cases
- Presentation – sixth decade
- Prognosis – usually good

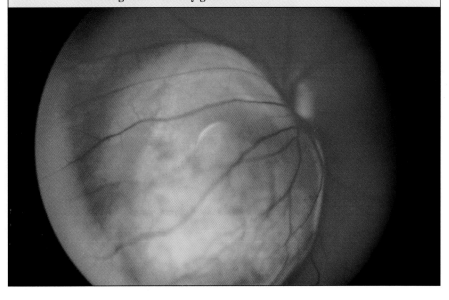

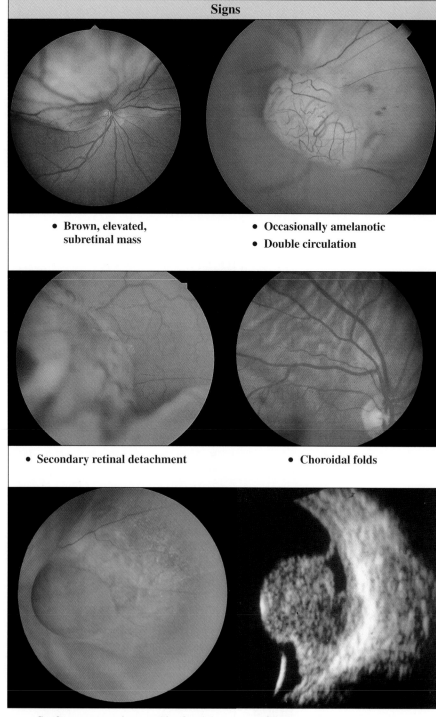

**Signs**

- Brown, elevated, subretinal mass

- Occasionally amelanotic
- Double circulation

- Secondary retinal detachment

- Choroidal folds

- Surface orange pigment (lipofuscin) is common
- Mushroom-shaped if breaks through Bruch's membrane

- Ultrasound – acoustic hollowness, choroidal excavation and orbital shadowing

## Differential diagnosis

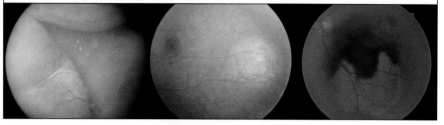

- Large choroidal naevus
- Metastatic tumour
- Localized choroidal haemangioma

- Choroidal detachment
- Choroidal granuloma
- Dense subretinal or sub-RPE haemorrhage

## TREATMENT OPTIONS

1. Brachytherapy
   – less than 10 mm elevation and 20 mm diameter
2. Charged particle irradiation
   – if unsuitable for brachytherapy
3. Transpupillary thermotherapy
   – selected small tumours
4. Trans-scleral local resection
   – carefully selected tumours less than 16 mm in diameter
5. Enucleation
   – very large tumours, particularly if useful vision lost
6. Exenteration
   – extraocular extension

| Histological classification | |
| --- | --- |
| 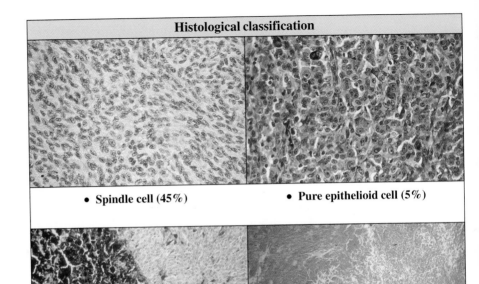 | |
| • Spindle cell (45%) | • Pure epithelioid cell (5%) |
| • Mixed cell (45%) | • Necrotic (5%) |

## POOR PROGNOSTIC FACTORS

1. Histological
   - Epithelioid cells
   - Closed vascular loops
   - Lymphocytic infiltration
2. Large size
3. Extrascleral extension
4. Anterior location
5. Age over 65 years

5. Choroidal naevus

**Typical naevus**

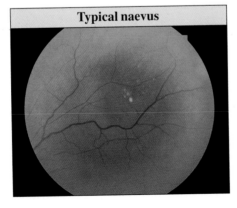

- Common – 2% of population
- Round slate-grey with indistinct margins
- Surface drusen
- Flat or slightly elevated
- Diameter less than 5 mm
- Location – anywhere
- Asymptomatic

## Suspicious naevus

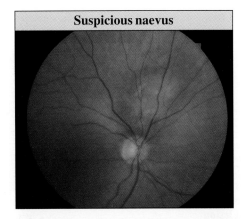

- Diameter more than 5 mm
- Elevation 2 mm or more
- Surface lipofuscin
- Posterior margin within 3 mm of disc
- May have symptoms due to serous fluid

## 6. Choroidal haemangioma

### Circumscribed

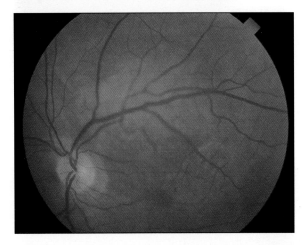

- Presentation – adult life
- Dome-shaped or placoid, red-orange mass
- Commonly at posterior pole
- Between 3 and 9 mm in diameter
- May blanch with external globe pressure
- Surface cystoid retinal degeneration
- Exudative retinal detachment
- Treatment – radiotherapy if vision threatened

### Diffuse

- Typically affects patients with Sturge–Weber syndrome

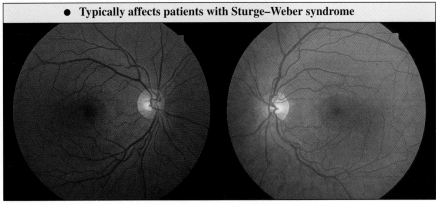

- Can be missed unless compared with normal fellow eye as shown here
- Diffuse thickening, most marked at posterior pole

## 7. Choroidal metastatic carcinoma

● Most frequent primary site is breast in women and bronchus in men

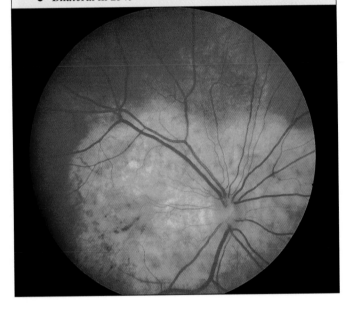

● Fast-growing, creamy-white, placoid lesion
● Most frequently at posterior pole

● Deposits may be multiple
● Bilateral in 10–30%

## 8. Choroidal osseous choristoma

● Very rare, benign, slow-growing ossifying tumour
● Typically affects young women
● Orange-yellow, oval lesion
● Well-defined, scalloped, geographical borders
● Most commonly peripapillary or at posterior pole
● Diffuse mottling of RPE
● Bilateral in 25%

## 9. Melanocytoma

- Affects dark-skinned individuals
- Usually asymptomatic
- Most frequently affects optic nerve head
- Black lesion with feathery edges

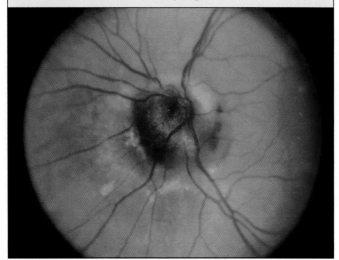

# RETINOBLASTOMA

1. **Important facts**

2. **Presentation**

3. **Signs**
   - Endophytic
   - Exophytic

4. **Treatment**

5. **Poor prognostic factors**

6. **Histology**

7. **Differential diagnosis of leukocoria**

1. Most common primary, malignant, intraocular tumour of childhood (1:20 000)
2. No sexual predilection
3. Presents before age of 3 years (average 3 months)
4. Heritable (40%) or non-heritable (60%)
5. Predisposing gene (RPE 1) on 13q14

2. Presentations

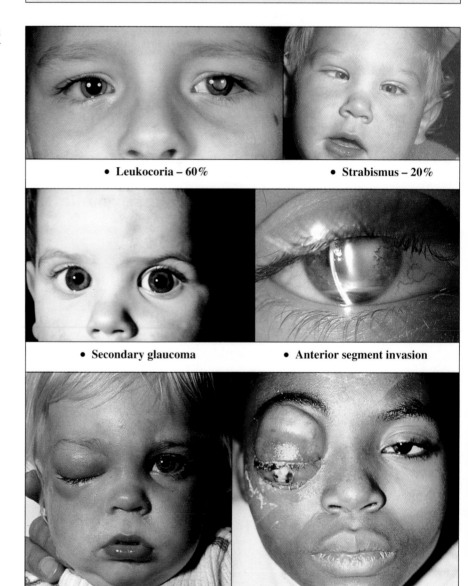

* Leukocoria – 60%  •  Strabismus – 20%

* Secondary glaucoma  •  Anterior segment invasion

* Orbital inflammation  •  Orbital invasion

## 3. Signs

**Endophytic**

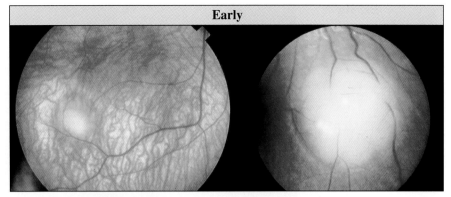

- White flat lesion
- Placoid lesion

More advanced

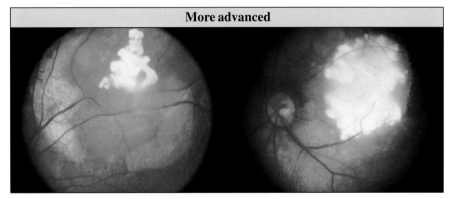

- Friable white mass
- Cottage cheese appearance

Late

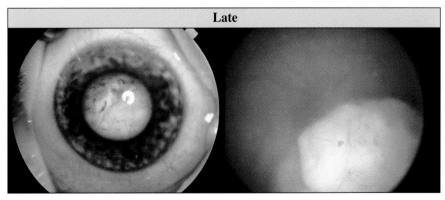

- Fine surface blood vessels
- Vitreous seedings

**Exophytic**

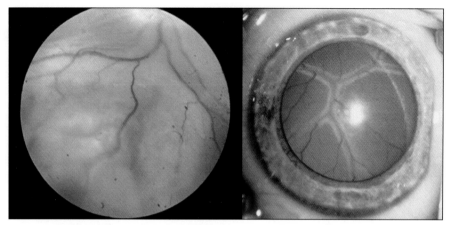

- Multiglobulated white mass with overlying retinal detachment
- May be difficult to visualize through deep detachment

**4. Treatment**

1. Small tumours
   - Laser photocoagulation
   - Transpupillary thermotherapy
   - Cryotherapy
2. Medium tumours
   - Brachytherapy
   - Chemotherapy
   - External beam radiotherapy
3. Large tumours
   - Chemotherapy followed by local treatment
   - Enucleation
4. Extraocular extension
   - External beam radiotherapy
5. Metastatic disease
   - Chemotherapy

**5. Poor prognostic factors**

1. Optic nerve involvement
2. Choroidal invasion
3. Large tumour
4. Anterior location
5. Poor cellular differentiation
6. Older children

## 6. Histology

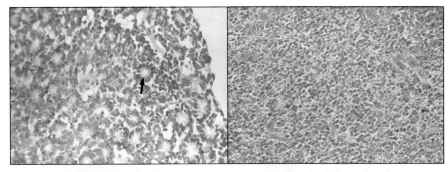

- Well-differentiated with many Flexner–Wintersteiner rosettes
- Poorly differentiated

## 7. Differential diagnosis of leukocoria

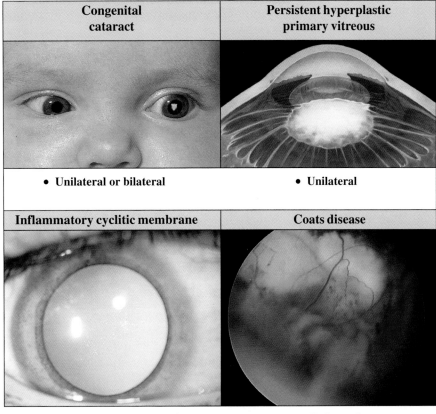

| Congenital cataract | Persistent hyperplastic primary vitreous |
|---|---|
| • Unilateral or bilateral | • Unilateral |
| Inflammatory cyclitic membrane | Coats disease |
| • Unilateral or bilateral | • Unilateral |

| Posterior pole toxocara granuloma | Advanced retinopathy of prematurity |
|---|---|
| 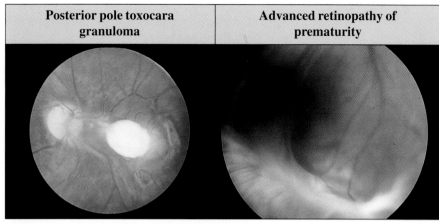 | |
| • Unilateral | • Always bilateral but may be asymmetrical |

# PATHOGENESIS AND SIGNS OF RETINAL DETACHMENT (RD)

1. **Rhegmatogenous RD**
   - Fresh
   - Longstanding
   - Proliferative vitreoretinopathy

2. **Diabetic tractional RD**

3. **Exudative RD**

4. **Differential diagnosis of RD**

## 1. Rhegmato-genous RD

| Pathogenesis |
|---|
| **Two components for retinal break formation** |
| ● Acute PVD |
| ● Predisposing peripheral retinal degeneration |
| **Possible sequelae of acute PVD** |

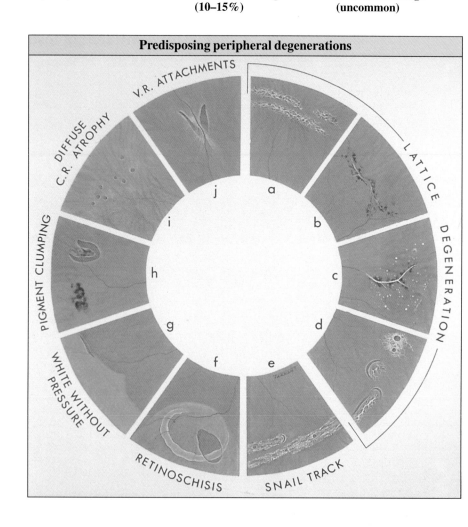

- ● Uncomplicated PVD (85%)
- ● Retinal tear formation and haemorrhage (10–15%)
- ● Avulsion of retinal vessel and haemorrhage (uncommon)

**Predisposing peripheral degenerations**

V.R. ATTACHMENTS

DIFFUSE C.R. ATROPHY

LATTICE DEGENERATION

PIGMENT CLUMPING

WHITE WITHOUT PRESSURE

RETINOSCHISIS

SNAIL TRACK

a
b
c
d
e
f
g
h
i
j

**Fresh**

| Signs |
|---|
| • Annual incidence – 1:10 000 of population |
| • Eventually bilateral in 10% |

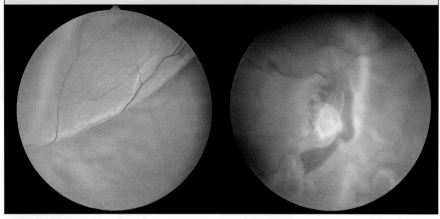

• Convex, deep mobile elevation extending to ora serrata
• Slightly opaque with dark blood vessels

• Loss of choroidal pattern
• Retinal breaks

**Longstanding**

| Signs |
|---|

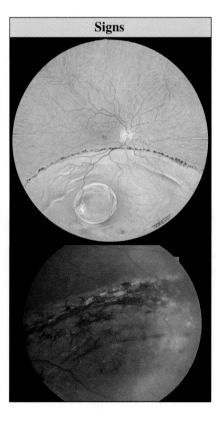

• Frequently inferior with small holes
• Very thin retina
• Secondary intraretinal cysts

• Demarcation lines (high-water marks)

**Proliferative vitreoretinopathy**

| Grade A (minimal) | Grade B (moderate) | Grade C (severe) |
|---|---|---|
| 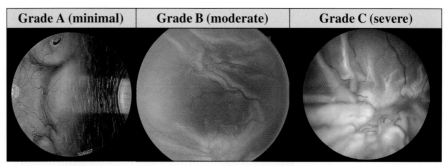 | | |
| • Vitreous haze and tobacco dust | • Retinal wrinkling and stiffness<br>• Rolled edges of tears | • Rigid retinal folds<br>• Vitreous condensations and strands |

2. Diabetic tractional RD

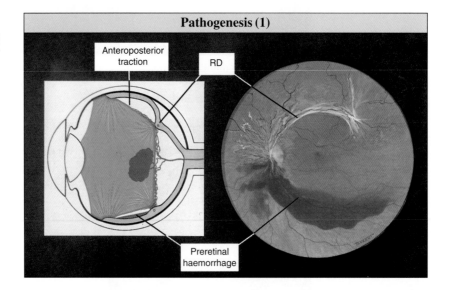

Pathogenesis (1)

Anteroposterior traction

RD

Preretinal haemorrhage

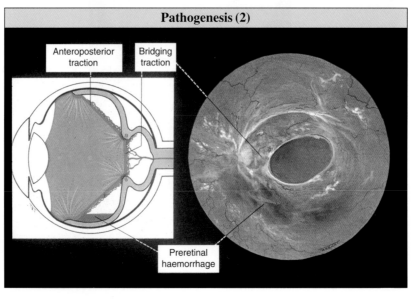

Pathogenesis (2)

Anteroposterior traction

Bridging traction

Preretinal haemorrhage

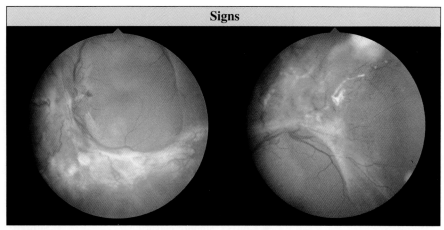

- Concave, shallow immobile elevation
- Highest at sites of vitreoretinal traction
- Slow progression and variable fibrosis
- Does not extend to ora serrata

**3. Exudative RD**

## PATHOGENESIS AND CAUSES

- Damage to RPE by subretinal disease
- Passage of fluid derived from choroid into subretinal space
    1. Choroidal tumours
        - Primary
        - Metastatic
    2. Intraocular inflammation
        - Harada disease
        - Posterior scleritis
    3. Systemic
        - Toxaemia of pregnancy
        - Hypoproteinaemia
    4. Iatrogenic
        - RD surgery
        - Excessive retinal photocoagulation
    5. Miscellaneous
        - Choroidal neovascularization
        - Uveal effusion syndrome

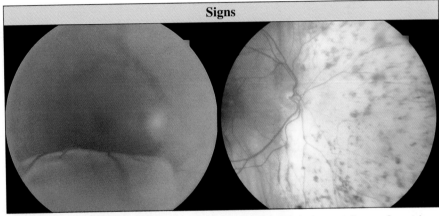

- Convex, smooth elevation
- May be very mobile and deep with shifting fluid

- Subretinal pigment (leopard spots) after flattening

## 4. Differential diagnosis of RD

| Degenerative retinoschisis | Choroidal detachment |
|---|---|

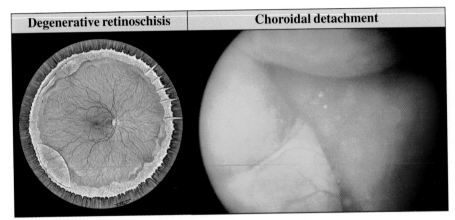

- Frequently bilateral
- Smooth, thin and immobile
- Occasionally breaks in one or both layers

- Associated with hypotony
- Unilateral, brown, smooth, solid and immobile
- Ora serrata may be visible

# PRINCIPLES OF RETINAL DETACHMENT SURGERY

1. **Scleral buckling**
   - Configuration of buckles
   - Preliminary steps
   - Localization of breaks
   - Cryotherapy
   - Insertion of local explant
   - Encircling procedure
   - Drainage of subretinal fluid
   - Causes of early failure

2. **Pneumatic retinopexy**

3. **Vitrectomy**
   - Giant tears
   - Proliferative vitreoretinopathy
   - Diabetic tractional RD

## 1. Scleral buckling

**Configuration of buckles**

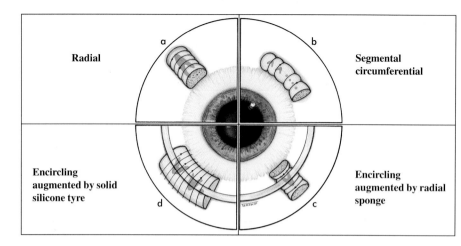

Radial

a

Segmental circumferential

b

Encircling augmented by solid silicone tyre

d

c

Encircling augmented by radial sponge

**Preliminary steps**

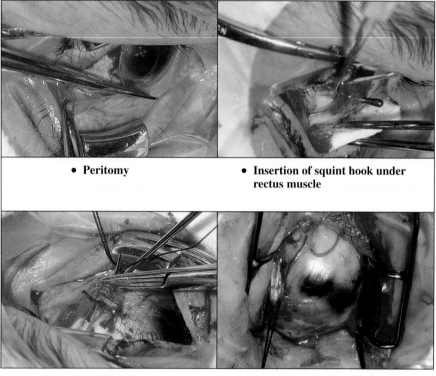

- Peritomy
- Insertion of squint hook under rectus muscle
- Insertion of bridle suture
- Inspection of sclera for thinning or anomalous vortex veins

**Localization of breaks**

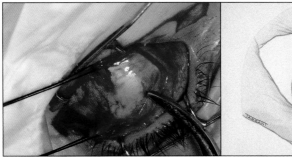

- Insert 5/0 Dacron scleral suture at site of apex of break
- Grasp cut suture with curved mosquito forceps close to knot

- While viewing with indirect ophthalmoscope check position of indentation in relation to break

**Cryotherapy**

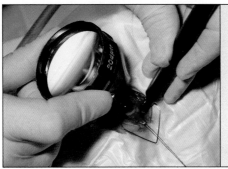
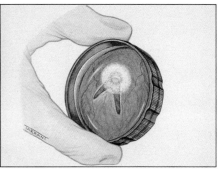

- While viewing with indirect ophthalmoscope indent sclera gently with tip of cryoprobe

- Freeze break until sensory retina just turns white

**Insertion of local explant**

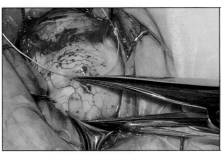
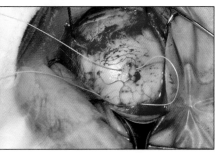

- Distance separating sutures measured and marked

- Insertion of mattress-type suture

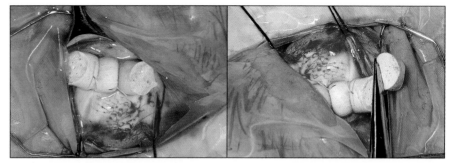

- Sutures tightened over explant
- Ends trimmed

**Encircling procedure**

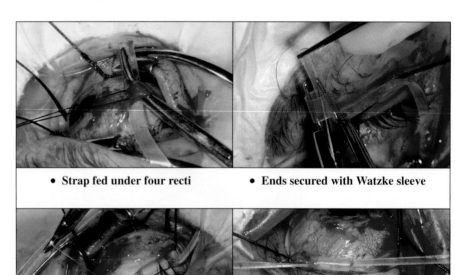

- Strap fed under four recti
- Ends secured with Watzke sleeve

- Strap slid posteriorly and secured in each quadrant
- Strap tightened to produce required amount of internal indentation

**Drainage of subretinal fluid**

| Indications |
|---|
| ● **Difficulty in localizing break** |
| ● **Immobile retina** |
| ● **Longstanding RD** |
| ● **Inferior RD** |

| Technique |
|---|

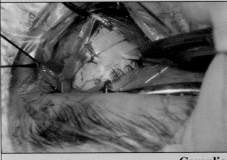 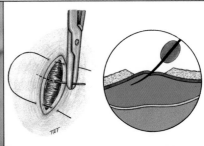

| Complications |
|---|

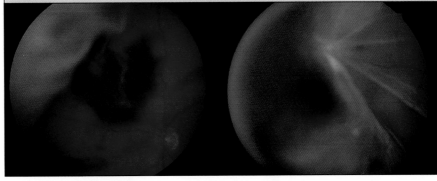

| ● **Haemorrhage** | ● **Retinal incarceration** |
|---|---|

**Causes of early failure**

| Buckle failure |
|---|

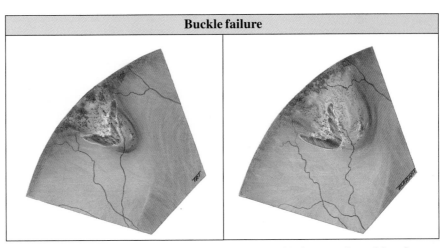

| ● **Buckle inadequate size or height** | ● **Buckle incorrectly positioned** |
|---|---|

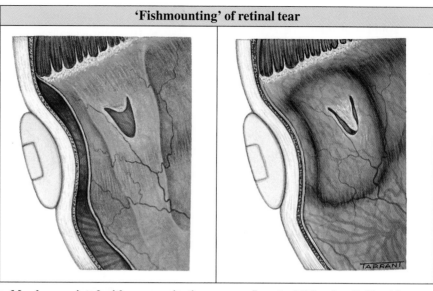

- May be associated with communicating radial retinal fold

- Insert additional radial buckle

## 2. Pneumatic retinopexy

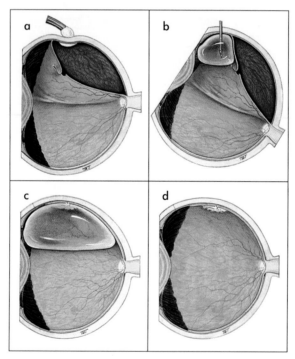

*Indications*
- RD with superior breaks

*Technique*
- Cryotherapy (a)
- Gas injection (b)
- Postoperative positioning (c)
- Flat retina (d)

## 3. Vitrectomy

### Giant tears

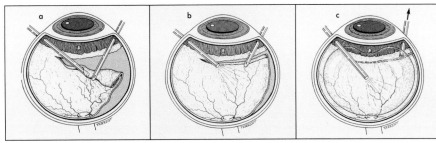

- Unrolling of flap with light pipe and probe
- Completion of unrolling
- Injection of silicone oil or heavy liquid

### Proliferative vitreo-retinopathy

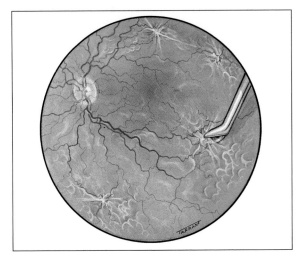

- Dissection of star folds and peeling of membranes
- Injection of expanding gas or silicone oil

### Diabetic tractional RD

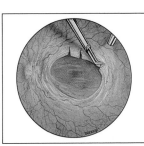 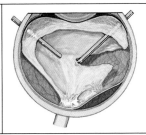 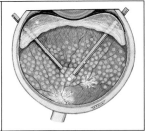

- Release of circumferential traction
- Release of antero-posterior traction
- Endophotocoagulation

# AGE-RELATED MACULAR DEGENERATION (AMD)

1. Drusen

2. Drusen and AMD

3. Atrophic AMD

4. Exudative AMD
   - Pigment epithelial detachment
   - Choroidal neovascularization

## 1. Drusen

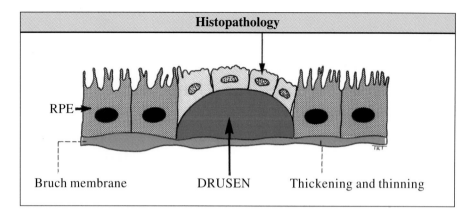

**Histopathology**

RPE

Bruch membrane · DRUSEN · Thickening and thinning

| Signs | |
|---|---|
| **Hard** | **Soft** |

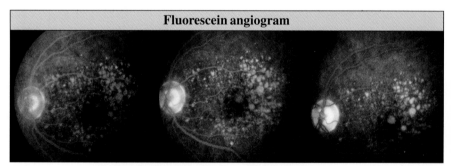

- **Small well-defined spots**
- **Usually innocuous**

- **Larger, ill-defined spots**
- **May enlarge and coalesce**
- **Increased risk of AMD**

**Fluorescein angiogram**

Degree of hyperfluorescence depends on:
- **Extent of overlying RPE atrophy (window defect)**
- **Amount of staining**
- **Lipid content**

**2. Drusen and AMD**

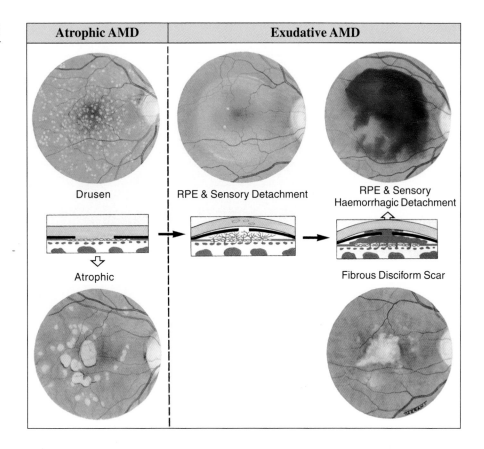

| Atrophic AMD | Exudative AMD |
|---|---|

Drusen

RPE & Sensory Detachment

RPE & Sensory Haemorrhagic Detachment

Atrophic

Fibrous Disciform Scar

**3. Atrophic AMD**

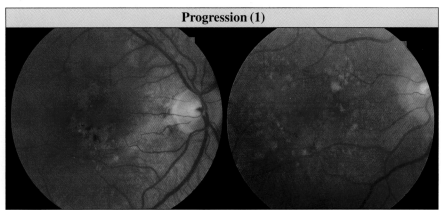

Progression (1)

- **Initially drusen and non-specific RPE changes**

### Progression (2)

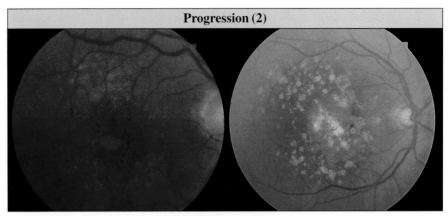

- Later geographic atrophy

| Fluorescein angiogram | Management |
|---|---|

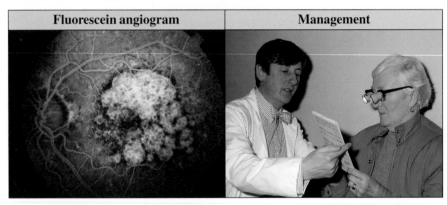

| • Hyperfluorescence from RPE window defect | • Low-vision aids if appropriate |

## 4. Exudative AMD

**Pigment epithelial detachment (PED)**

### Signs of PED

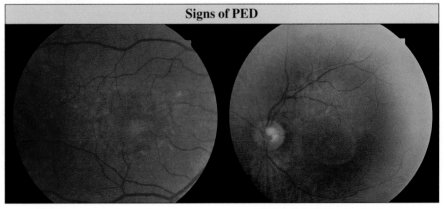

| • Circumscribed, dome-shaped elevation | • Sub-RPE fluid may be clear or turbid |

## Fluorescein angiogram of PED

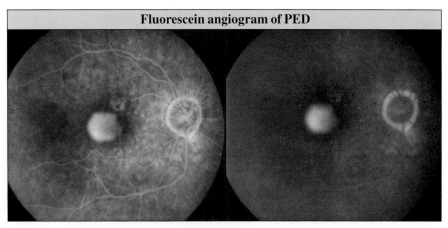

- Progressive increase in *hyper*fluorescence but not in size

## ICG angiogram of PED

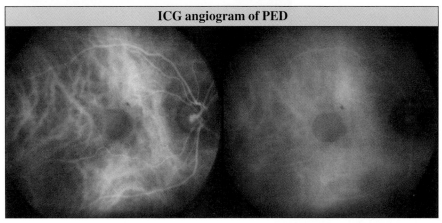

- Early, well-defined *hypo*fluorescence

- Later, thin surrounding *hyper*fluorescent ring but no increase in size

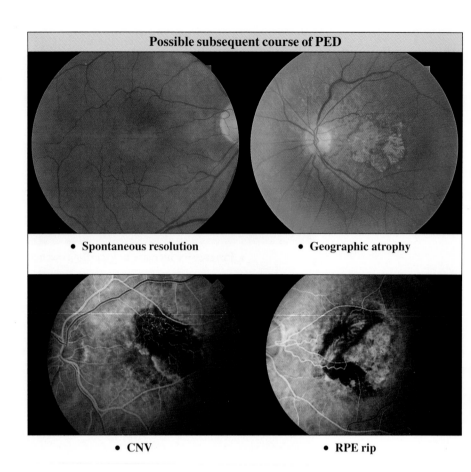

**Possible subsequent course of PED**

- Spontaneous resolution
- Geographic atrophy
- CNV
- RPE rip

**Choroidal neovascularization (CNV)**

- Less common than atrophic AMD but more serious
- Metamorphopsia is initial symptom
- Most lesions are not visible clinically

### Suspicious clinical signs of CNV

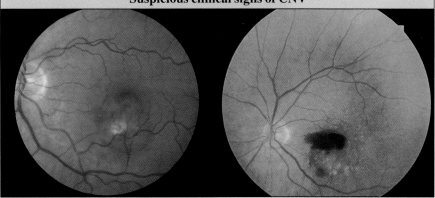

- Pinkish-yellow subretinal lesion with fluid
- Subretinal blood or lipid

### Angiographic classification of CNV

| Well-defined (classic) | Occult |
| --- | --- |

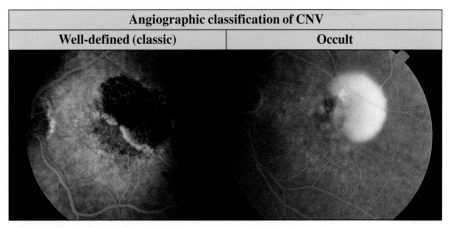

| Well-defined (classic) | Occult |
| --- | --- |
| • Extrafoveal > 200 µm from centre of FAZ<br>• Juxtafoveal < 200 µm from centre of FAZ<br>• Subfoveal – involving centre of FAZ | • Poorly defined<br>• Obscured by PED, blood or exudate |

| Classic |
| :---: |
| **Fluorescein angiogram of classic CNV** |

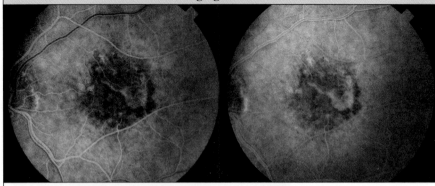

- Very early 'lacy' filling pattern
- Leakage into subretinal space and around CNV

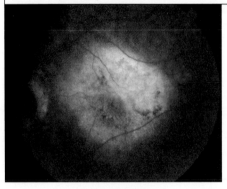

- Late staining

| ICG angiogram in PED with occult CNV |
| :---: |

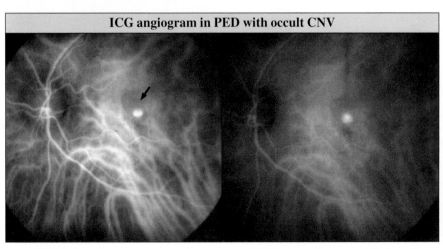

- PED is *hypo*fluorescent (arrow)
- CNV is *hyper*fluorescent (hot spot)

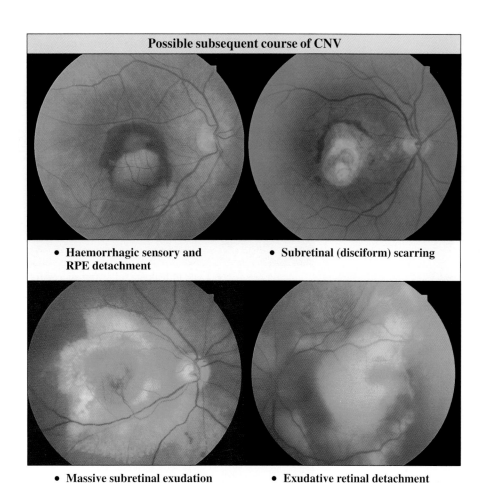

**Possible subsequent course of CNV**

- Haemorrhagic sensory and RPE detachment
- Subretinal (disciform) scarring
- Massive subretinal exudation
- Exudative retinal detachment

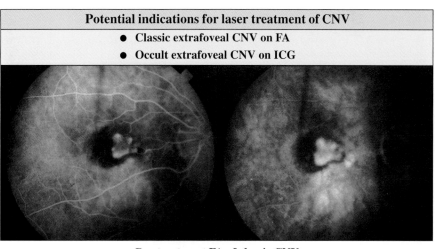

**Potential indications for laser treatment of CNV**

- Classic extrafoveal CNV on FA
- Occult extrafoveal CNV on ICG

- Pre-treatment FA of classic CNV

## Technique of laser photocoagulation of CNV

- Perimeter is treated with overlapping 200 μm (0.2–0.5 sec) burns
- Entire area is covered with high energy burns

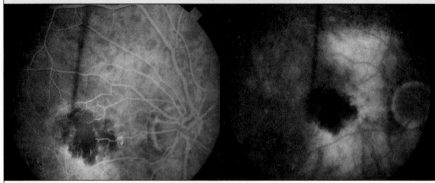

- Lack of leakage following successful treatment

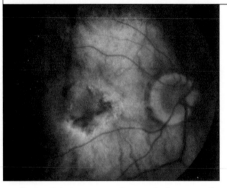

- Late staining around margin is normal

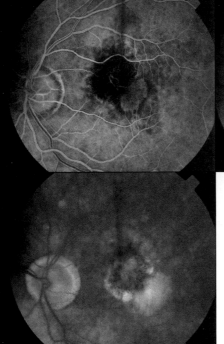

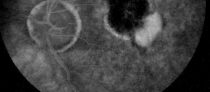

● Recurrence of CNV several months
  after initially successful treatment

# OTHER ACQUIRED MACULOPATHIES

1. **Central serous retinopathy**

2. **Idiopathic macular hole**

3. **Idiopathic premacular fibrosis**

4. **Cystoid macular oedema**

5. **Myopic maculopathy**

6. **Choroidal folds**

7. **Angioid streaks**

## 1. Central serous retinopathy

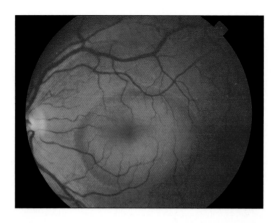

- Self-limiting disease of young or middle-aged men
- Usually unilateral
- Localized, shallow detachment of sensory retina at posterior pole
- Often outlined by glistening reflex

| Fluorescein angiogram (1) |
| :---: |
| **Smoke-stack appearance** |

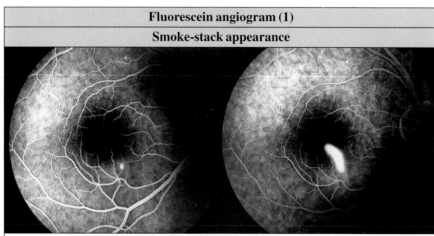

- Early hyperfluorescent spot
- Later dye passage into subretinal space and vertical ascent

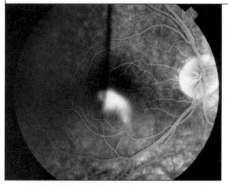

- Subsequent lateral spread until entire area filled

| Fluorescein angiogram (2) |
| :---: |
| **Ink-blot appearance – less common** |

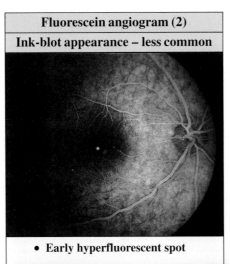

- **Early hyperfluorescent spot**

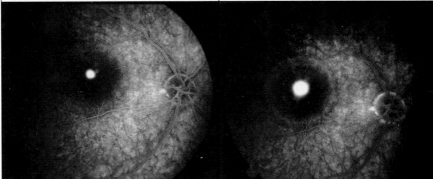

- **Subsequent concentric spread until entire area filled**

| Treatment |
| :---: |
| ● **Most cases are self-limiting and do not require treatment** |
| **Laser photocoagulation to RPE leak** |

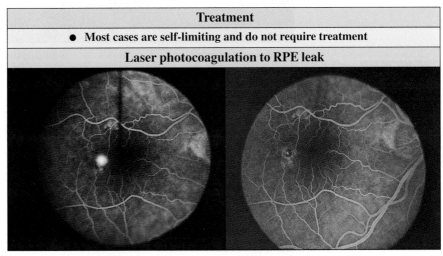

- **Pre-treatment**
- **Post-treatment**

- **4 months should elapse before considering treatment**
- **Treatment induces resolution and lowers recurrence rate**
- **Does not influence final visual outcome**

## 2. Idiopathic macular hole

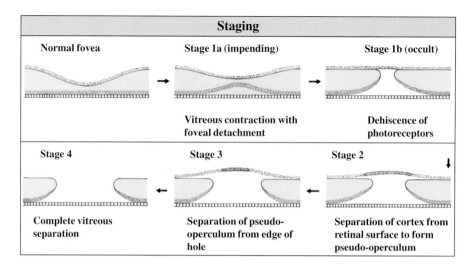

**Staging**

| Normal fovea | Stage 1a (impending) | Stage 1b (occult) |
|---|---|---|
| | Vitreous contraction with foveal detachment | Dehiscence of photoreceptors |

| Stage 4 | Stage 3 | Stage 2 |
|---|---|---|
| Complete vitreous separation | Separation of pseudo-operculum from edge of hole | Separation of cortex from retinal surface to form pseudo-operculum |

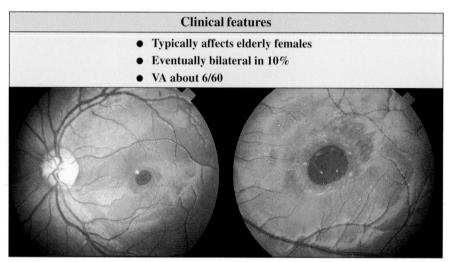

**Clinical features**

- Typically affects elderly females
- Eventually bilateral in 10%
- VA about 6/60

- Round punched-out area at fovea
- Surrounding halo of subretinal fluid
- Multiple yellow deposits within crater
- Positive Watzke–Allen sign

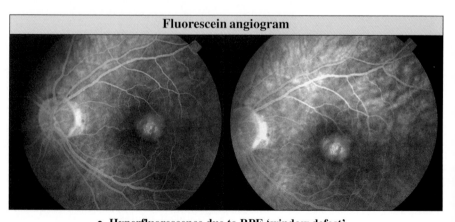

**Fluorescein angiogram**

- Hyperfluorescence due to RPE 'window defect'

## TREATMENT

1. **Indications**
   - **Full-thickness macular hole**
   - **Visual acuity < 6/18**
   - **Duration < 1 year**
2. **Technique**
   - **Vitrectomy and fluid–gas exchange**
3. **Results**
   - **Closure in about 60%**
   - **40% regain 2 or more lines of VA**

## 3. Idiopathic premacular fibrosis

**Cellophane maculopathy**

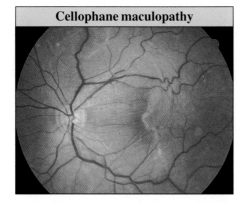

- **Translucent epiretinal membrane**
- **Fine retinal striae and mild vascular distortion**

**Macular pucker**

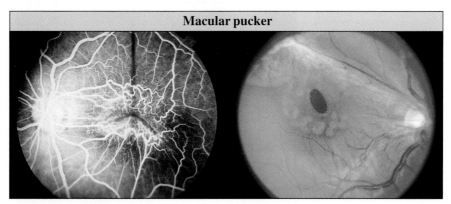

- **Severe retinal wrinkling and vascular distortion**
- **Pucker emanating from epicentre**

- **Opaque epiretinal membrane**
- **May be associated with macular pseudo-hole**

## 4. Cystoid macular oedema

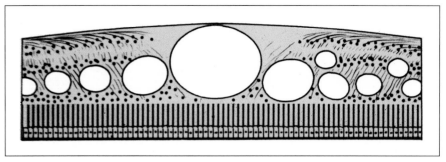

- Fluid-filled microcysts in outer plexiform and inner nuclear layer

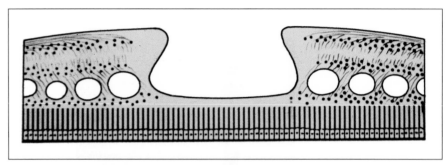

- May lead to lamellar hole formation if longstanding

**Important causes**

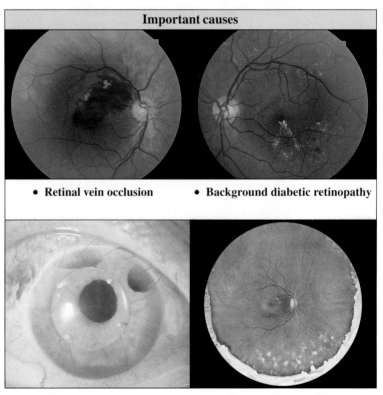

- Retinal vein occlusion
- Background diabetic retinopathy
- Post cataract surgery
- Intermediate uveitis

| Signs |
|---|

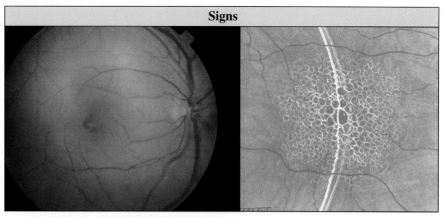

- Loss of foveal depression
- Yellow spot at foveola

- Retinal thickening
- Multiple cystoid areas

| Fluorescein angiogram |
|---|

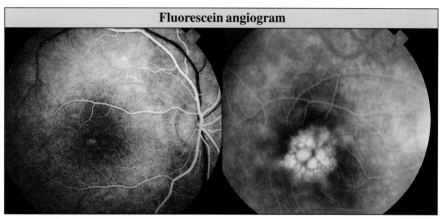

- Early parafoveal leakage

- Late pooling with 'flower-petal' pattern

5. Myopic maculopathy

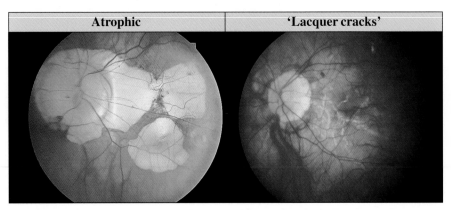

| Atrophic | 'Lacquer cracks' |
|---|---|

- Progressive chorioretinal atrophy
- May be associated with macular hole

- Large breaks in Bruch membrane
- Develop in about 5% of highly myopic eyes

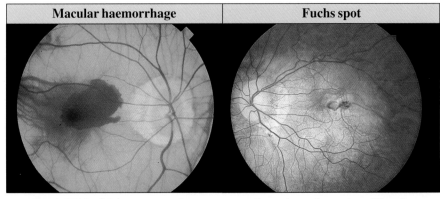

| Macular haemorrhage | Fuchs spot |
|---|---|

- From CNV with lacquer cracks
- From lacquer cracks alone

- Secondary pigment proliferation
- Follows absorption of blood

## Other fundus changes

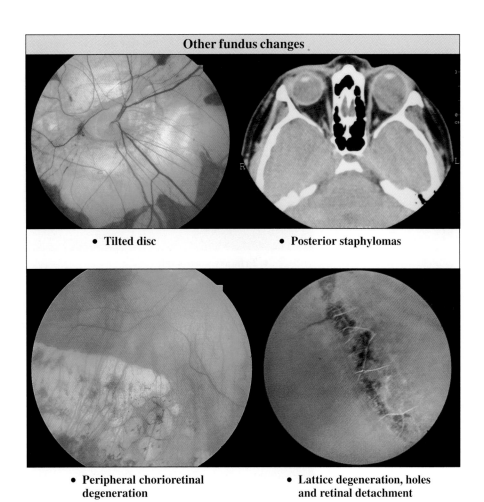

- Tilted disc
- Posterior staphylomas

- Peripheral chorioretinal degeneration
- Lattice degeneration, holes and retinal detachment

## Ocular associations (1)
### Cataract

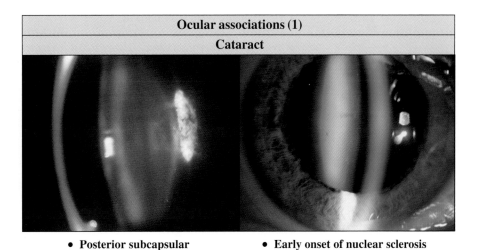

- Posterior subcapsular
- Early onset of nuclear sclerosis

| Ocular associations (2) |
|---|
| **Glaucoma** |

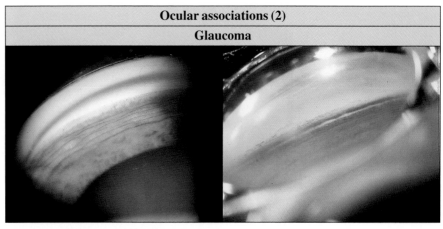

- Primary open-angle
- Pigmentary

## 6. Choroidal folds

| Signs | Fluorescein angiogram |
|---|---|

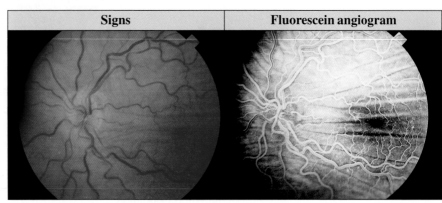

| Signs | Fluorescein angiogram |
|---|---|
| • Parallel, horizontal striae at posterior pole<br>• Occasionally vertical, oblique or irregular<br>• Trough is darker than crest | • Alternating hyperfluorescent and hypofluorescent streaks<br>• Trough is hypofluorescent – blocked background fluorescence<br>• Crest is hyperfluorescent – window defect |

| Causes (1) |
|---|

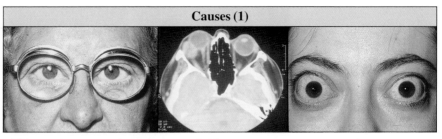

- Bilateral in hypermetropic patients
- Orbital mass
- Thyroid ophthalmopathy

| Causes (2) |
|---|

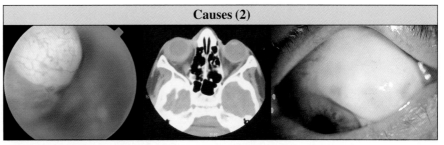

- Choroidal tumour
- Posterior scleritis
- Severe ocular hypotony

## 7. Angioid streaks

- **Bilateral, crack-like dehiscence in Bruch membrane**
- **Secondary changes in RPE and choriocapillaris**

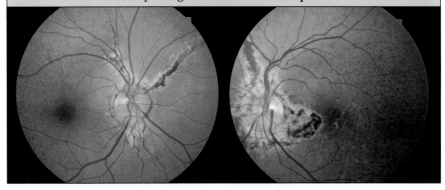

- Linear lesions with irregular serrated edges
- Radiate outwards from disc

- Eventually surround disc
- 'Peau d'orange' mottling of RPE particularly temporally

| Ocular associations |
|---|

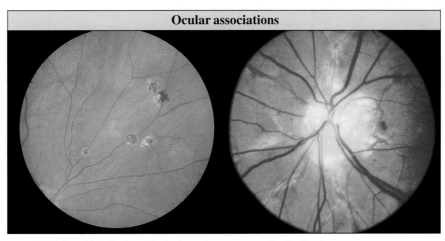

- Peripheral focal atrophic 'salmon' spots – common

- Optic disc drusen – uncommon

## Fluorescein angiogram

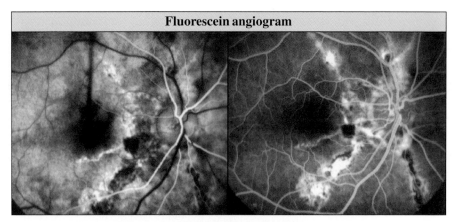

- Hyperfluorescence due to RPE window defects over streaks

## Complications

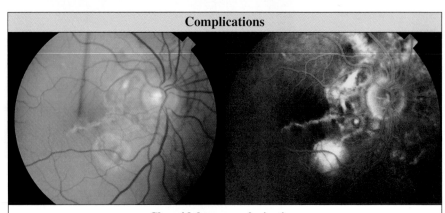

- Choroidal neovascularization

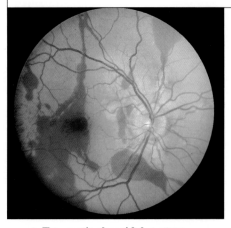

- Traumatic choroidal rupture

● **Present in approx. 50% of patients**

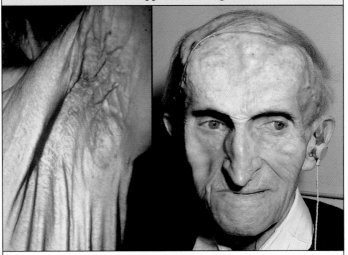

- **Pseudoxanthoma elasticum (most common)**
- **Paget disease (uncommon)**

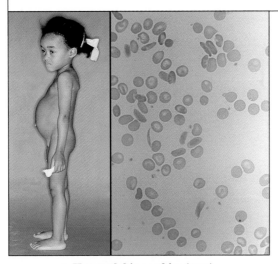

- **Haemoglobinopathies (rare)**

# HEREDITARY RETINAL DYSTROPHIES

## 1. Photoreceptor dystrophies
- Retinitis pigmentosa
- Retinitis punctata albescens
- Fundus albipunctatus
- Cone dystrophy
- Leber congenital amaurosis

## 2. Retinal pigment epithelial dystrophies
- Best vitelliform macular dystrophy
- Adult Best vitelliform macular dystrophy
- Stargardt macular dystrophy
- Fundus flavimaculatus
- Familial dominant drusen
- Sorsby pseudo-inflammatory macular dystrophy
- North Carolina macular dystrophy
- Butterfly macular dystrophy

## 1. Photoreceptor dystrophies

### Retinitis pigmentosa

---

### RETINITIS PIGMENTOSA

1. Inheritance
   - Sporadic (23%)
   - Dominant (43%)
   - Recessive (20%)
   - X-linked recessive (8%)
   - Uncertain (6%)
2. Presents – usually prior to 30 years
3. Prognosis – dominant worst, X-linked best
4. ERG – reduced

---

**Progression**

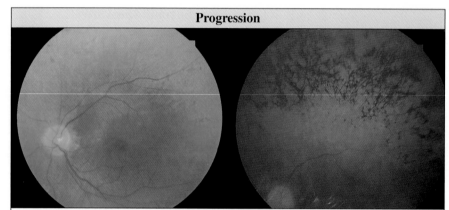

- Fine dust-like pigmentation
- Arteriolar attenuation

- Perivascular 'bone-spicule' pigmentation
- Initially mid-peripheral

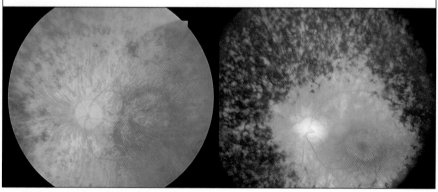

- Anterior and peripheral spread
- Unmasking of large choroidal vessels

- Optic disc pallor
- Maculopathy

## Ocular associations

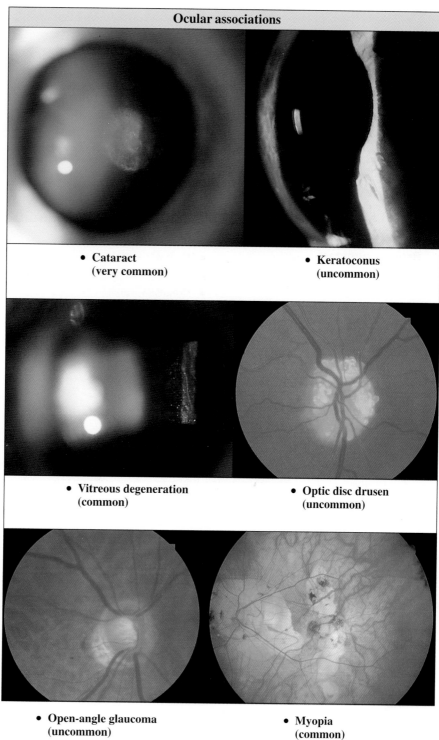

- Cataract
  (very common)

- Keratoconus
  (uncommon)

- Vitreous degeneration
  (common)

- Optic disc drusen
  (uncommon)

- Open-angle glaucoma
  (uncommon)

- Myopia
  (common)

| Atypical | |
|---|---|
| **Quadrantic** | **Sectorial** |

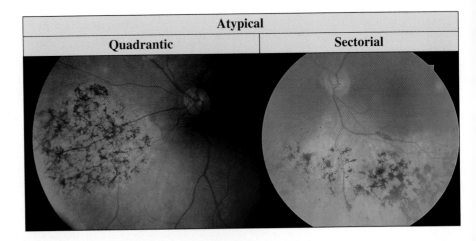

**Retinitis punctata albescens**

- Probably variant of retinitis pigmentosa
- Presents – usually under age 30 years
- Prognosis – poor
- ERG – reduced

- Scattered white dots extending from posterior pole to periphery
- Subsequent development of 'bone-spicule' pigmentation

**Fundus albipunctatus**

Inheritance – recessive

Congenital stationary night blindness

Prognosis – excellent

ERG – reduced

- Multitude of tiny yellow-white spots
- Extend from posterior pole to mid-periphery

- Fovea spared

**Cone dystrophy**

- Inheritance usually – sporadic, occasionally autosomal dominant or X-linked recessive
- Presents – first to third decade
- Prognosis – guarded
- ERG – reduced photopic, normal scotopic

**Progression**

- 'Bull's eye' macular lesion
- May be associated with golden tapetal reflex

- Later mild 'bone-spicule' pigmentation
- Very late geographic macular atrophy

**Leber congenital amaurosis**

- Inheritance – usually autosomal recessive
- Presentation – frequently perinatal
- Prognosis – very poor
- ERG – non-recordable

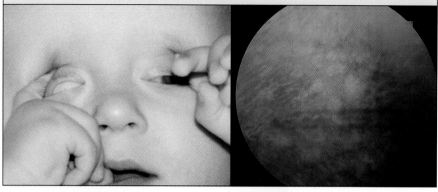

- Oculodigital syndrome
- Afferent pupillary defect

- Initially fundus may be normal
- Peripheral chorioretinal atrophy and granularity

## 2. Retinal pigment epithelial dystrophies

**Best vitelliform macular dystrophy**

- Inheritance – autosomal dominant
- Presents – first decade
- Signs – very variable
- Prognosis – guarded
- EOG – severely subnormal

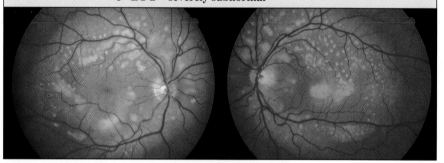

- Multifocal Best disease

## Stage 2

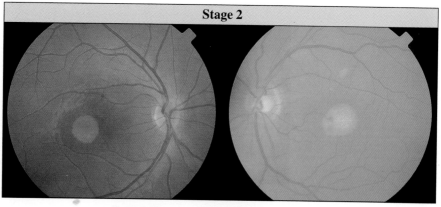

- During first to second decade
- 'Egg-yolk' or 'sunny-side-up' macular lesion
- VA – normal or slight decrease

## Fluorescein angiogram of stage 2

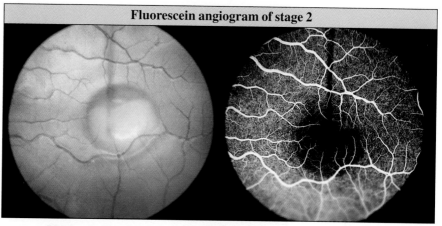

- Blockage of background choroidal fluorescence corresponding to lesion

## Stage 3

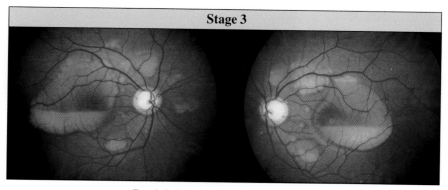

- Partial absorption and pseudohypopyon
- VA – slight decrease

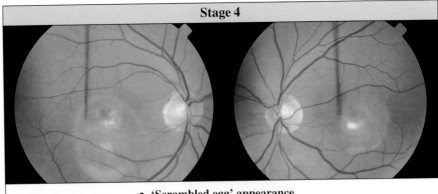

- 'Scrambled egg' appearance
- VA – moderate decrease

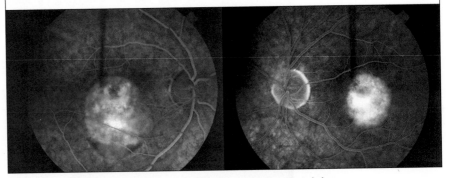

- FA shows hyperfluorescence due to staining

Stage 5

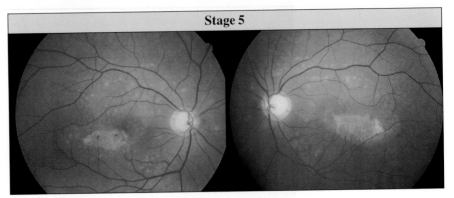

- Macular scar or atrophy
- VA – moderate to severe decrease

**Adult Best vitelliform macular dystrophy**

- Inheritance – dominant
- Presents – fourth to fifth decades, but may be asymptomatic
- Prognosis – usually good
- EOG – normal or slightly abnormal

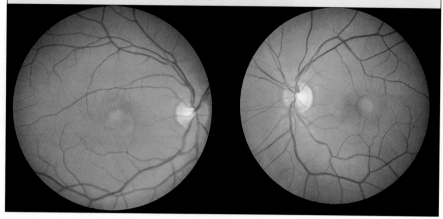

- Round or oval, slightly elevated, yellow, subfoveal lesion
- 1/3 to 1/2 disc diameter in size

**Stargardt macular dystrophy**

- Inheritance – usually recessive
- Presents – first to second decade
- Prognosis – poor
- ERG – reduced in advanced cases

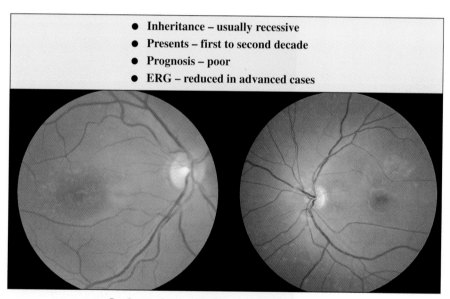

- Oval macular 'snail-slime' or 'beaten-bronze'
- Occasionally surrounded by yellow-white flecks

## End stage

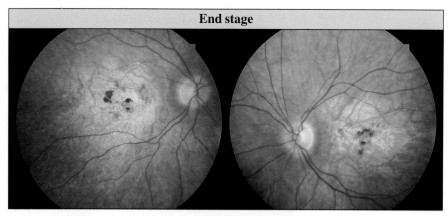

- Eventual atrophic maculopathy
- VA severe decrease

**Fundus flavimaculatus**

- Inheritance – usually recessive
- Presents – fourth to fifth decades
- Prognosis – good in most cases
- ERG – reduced in advanced cases

## Early stage

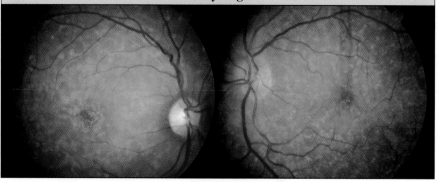

- Ill-defined, yellow-white flecks
- Extending from posterior pole to mid-periphery
- Vermilion colour fundus in about 50%

## Late stage

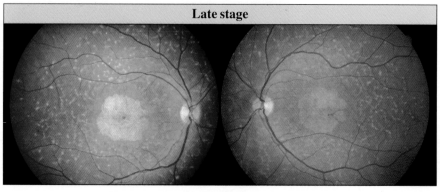

- Eventual atrophic maculopathy in some cases

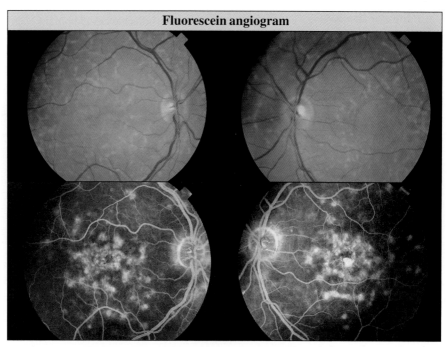

- Flecks are hyperfluorescent due to RPE atrophy
- Absence of normal background fluorescence (dark choroid)

**Familial dominant drusen**

- Presents – second to third decade, no symptoms
- Prognosis – usually good
- ERG – normal

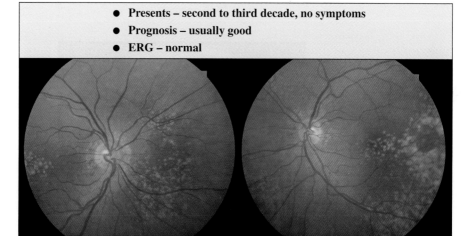

- Large, discrete, round, slightly raised, yellow lesions
- Usually symmetrical distribution
- Mainly at macula and peripapillary

**Sorsby pseudo-inflammatory macular dystrophy**

- Inheritance – dominant
- Presents – second to fourth decade
- Prognosis – very poor
- ERG – normal

**Progression**

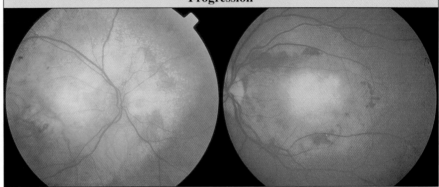

- Yellow-white confluent spots
- Along arcades and nasal to disc

- Eventual CNV and exudative maculopathy

**North Carolina macular dystrophy**

- Inheritance – dominant
- Presents – second decade
- Prognosis – variable
- ERG – normal

**Early stage**

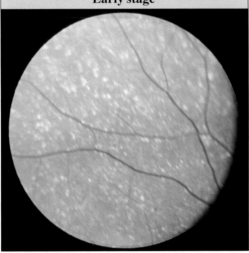

- Yellow-white spots at periphery and macula

## Progression

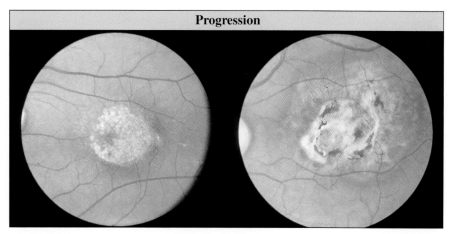

- Confluence of macular lesions

- Exudative or atrophic maculopathy

**Butterfly macular dystrophy**

- Inheritance – usually dominant
- Presents – fourth to fifth decades
- Prognosis – usually good
- ERG – normal

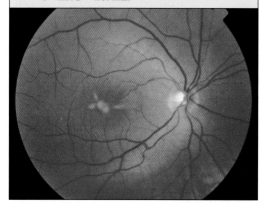

- Yellow pigment at fovea arranged in triradiate pattern

# HEREDITARY CHOROIDAL DYSTROPHIES

1. Choroideremia

2. Gyrate atrophy

3. Central areolar choroidal dystrophy

4. Diffuse choroidal atrophy

## 1. Choroid-eremia

- Inheritance – X-linked recessive
- Presents – first decade with nyctalopia
- Prognosis – good VA until late
- ERG – reduced

### Progression

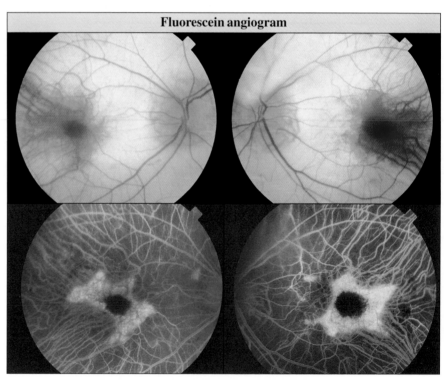

- Circumscribed atrophy of RPE and choroid
- Starting in periphery

- Gradual central spread
- Fovea spared until late

### Fluorescein angiogram

- Normal retinal vasculature
- Diffuse loss of choriocapillaris
- Preservation of larger choroidal vessels
- Hypofluorescence at fovea due to preservation of RPE
- Surrounding irregular hyperfluorescence due to preservation of choriocapillaris and partial loss of RPE

- Central patchy atrophy and mottling of RPE
- Peripheral diffuse pigmentary granularity

## 2. Gyrate atrophy

- Cause – deficiency of ornithine keto-acid aminotransferase
- Inheritance – autosomal recessive
- Presents – first decade with axial myopia and nyctalopia
- Prognosis – usually good VA until late
- ERG – severely reduced

**Progression**

- Mid-peripheral, circular patches of chorioretinal atrophy
- Enlargement and confluence

- Central and peripheral spread
- Late retinal vascular attenuation
- Fovea spared until late

## 3. Central areolar choroidal dystrophy

- Inheritance – dominant
- Presents – fifth decade
- Prognosis – poor
- ERG – normal

- Bilateral, circumscribed, atrophic maculopathy
- Prominent large choroidal vessels

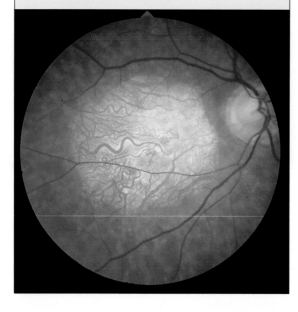

## 4. Diffuse choroidal atrophy

- Inheritance – dominant
- Presents – fourth to fifth decades
- Prognosis – poor
- ERG – reduced

- Diffuse atrophy of RPE and choriocapillaris
- Prominent large choroidal vessels

# HEREDITARY VITREORETINAL DEGENERATIONS

1. **Stickler syndrome**

2. **Congenital retinoschisis**

3. **Favre–Goldmann syndrome**

4. **Familial exudative vitreoretinopathy**

## 1. Stickler syndrome

- Inheritance – dominant
- Presents – first decade
- Prognosis – RD in 30%

| Vitreous | Retina |
| --- | --- |
| 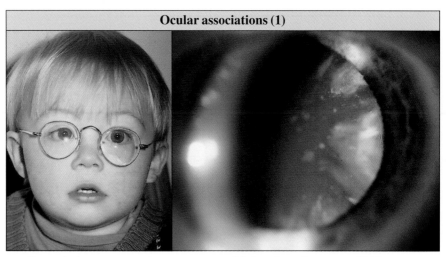 | |

- Empty central cavity
- Membranes extending into cavity

- Radial lattice-like degeneration
- RPE hyperplasia

### Ocular associations (1)

- Congenital non-progressive high myopia (85%)

- Wedge-shaped cataract (40%)

## Ocular associations (2)

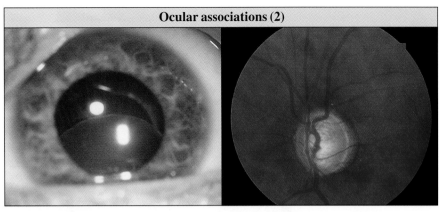

- Ectopia lentis (10%)      • Glaucoma (10%)

## Systemic features

| Facial anomalies | Arthropathy |
| --- | --- |

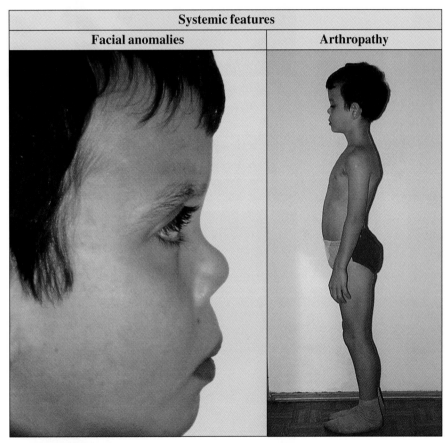

- Depressed nasal bridge and midfacial hypoplasia
- Micrognathia, glossoptosis and cleft palate

- Kyphoscoliosis
- Joint hyperflexibility
- Peripheral arthropathy

## 2. Congenital retinoschisis

- Inheritance – X-linked
- Presents – first decade with maculopathy
- Prognosis – poor (maculopathy, vitreous haemorrhage)
- ERG – decreased b-wave

| Maculopathy (100%) | Retinoschisis (50%) |
|---|---|

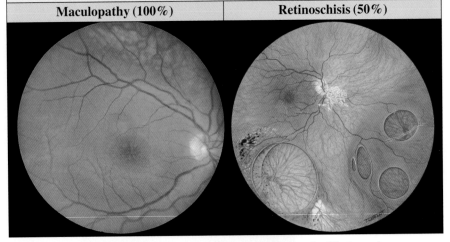

| | |
|---|---|
| • 'Bicycle-wheel' striae<br>• Eventually atrophic | • Extremely thin inner layer<br>• Round inner layer defects |

## 3. Favre–Goldmann syndrome

- Inheritance – recessive
- Presents – first decade with nyctalopia
- Prognosis – poor
- ERG – reduced

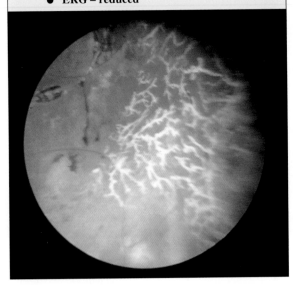

- Vitreous liquefaction
- Retinoschisis
- Pigmentary retinopathy
- White, dendritiform, arborescent peripheral lesions

## 4. Familial exudative vitreoretino-pathy

- Inheritance – dominant
- Presents – infancy
- Prognosis – poor (RD, vitreous haemorrhage and cataract)

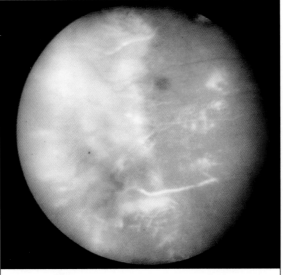

- Temporal fibrovascular proliferation similar to ROP

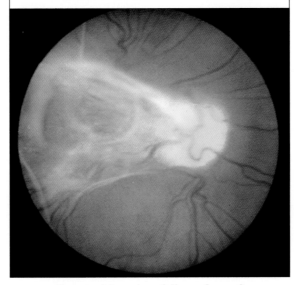

- Temporal dragging of disc and macula

# DIABETIC RETINOPATHY

1. **Adverse risk factors**

2. **Pathogenesis**

3. **Background diabetic retinopathy**

4. **Diabetic maculopathies**
   - Focal
   - Diffuse
   - Ischaemic

5. **Clinically significant macular oedema**

6. **Preproliferative diabetic retinopathy**

7. **Proliferative diabetic retinopathy**

1. **Adverse risk factors**

1. **Long duration of diabetes**
2. **Poor metabolic control**
3. **Pregnancy**
4. **Hypertension**
5. **Renal disease**
6. **Other**
   - **Obesity**
   - **Hyperlipidaemia**
   - **Smoking**
   - **Anaemia**

2. **Pathogenesis**

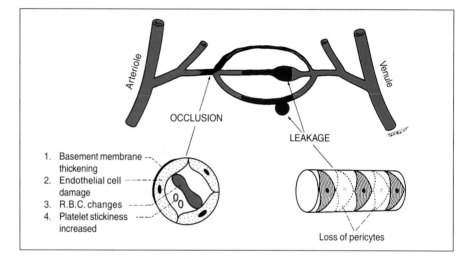

1. Basement membrane thickening
2. Endothelial cell damage
3. R.B.C. changes
4. Platelet stickiness increased

OCCLUSION

LEAKAGE

Arteriole

Venule

Loss of pericytes

**Consequences of retinal ischaemia**

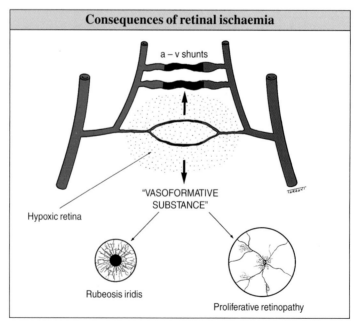

a – v shunts

Hypoxic retina

"VASOFORMATIVE SUBSTANCE"

Rubeosis iridis

Proliferative retinopathy

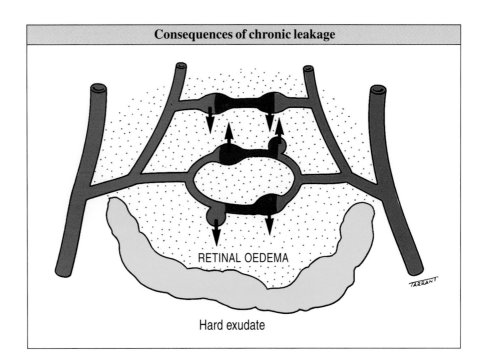

**Consequences of chronic leakage**

RETINAL OEDEMA

Hard exudate

### 3. Background diabetic retinopathy

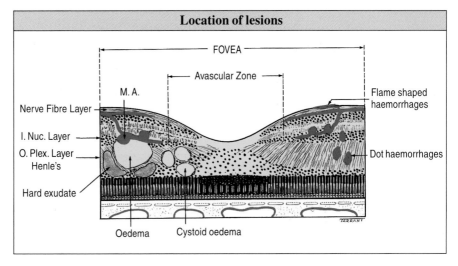

**Location of lesions**

FOVEA

Avascular Zone

M. A.

Nerve Fibre Layer

I. Nuc. Layer

O. Plex. Layer
Henle's

Hard exudate

Flame shaped
haemorrhages

Dot haemorrhages

Oedema    Cystoid oedema

| Signs |
|---|

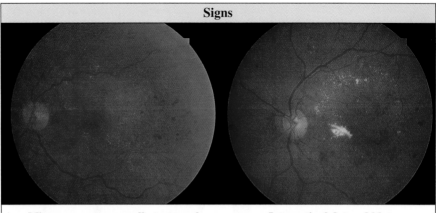

- Microaneurysms usually temporal to fovea
- Intraretinal dot and blot haemorrhages

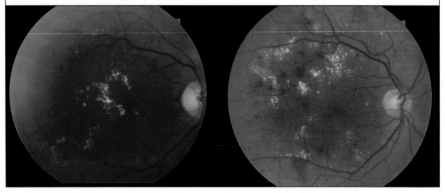

- Hard exudates frequently arranged in clumps or rings
- Retinal oedema seen as thickening on biomicroscopy

## 4. Diabetic maculopathies

### Focal

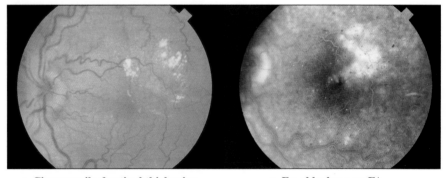

- Circumscribed retinal thickening
- Associated complete or incomplete circinate hard exudates

- Focal leakage on FA
- Focal photocoagulation
- Good prognosis

**Diffuse**

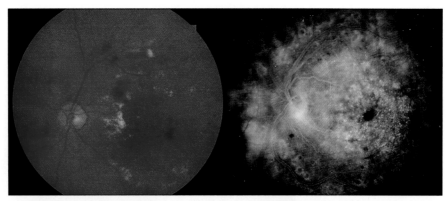

- Diffuse retinal thickening
- Frequent cystoid macular oedema
- Variable impairment of visual acuity

- Generalized leakage on FA
- Grid photocoagulation
- Guarded prognosis

**Ischaemic**

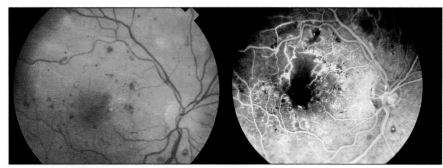

- Macula appears relatively normal
- Poor visual acuity

- Capillary non-perfusion on FA
- Treatment not appropriate

**5. Clinically significant macular oedema**

- Retinal oedema within 500 μm of centre of fovea

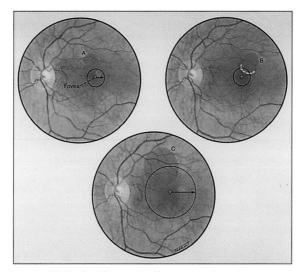

- Hard exudates within 500 μm of centre of fovea with adjacent oedema which may be outside 500 μm limit

- Retinal oedema one disc area or larger, any part of which is within one disc diameter (1500 μm) of centre of fovea

| Treatment | |
|---|---|
| **Grid treatment** | **Focal treatment** |

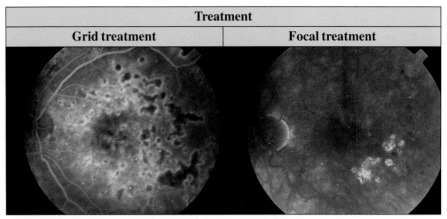

- For diffuse retinal thickening located more than 500 μm from centre of fovea and 500 μm from temporal margin of disc
- Gentle burns (100–200 μm, 0.10 sec), one burn width apart

- For microaneurysms in centre of hard exudate rings located 500–3000 μm from centre of fovea
- Gentle whitening or darkening of microaneurysm (100–200 μm, 0.10 sec)

## 6. Preproliferative diabetic retinopathy

| Signs |
|---|

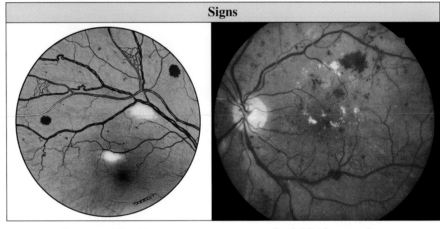

- Cotton-wool spots
- Venous irregularities

- Dark blot haemorrhages
- Intraretinal microvascular abnormalities

*Treatment* — Not required but watch for proliferative disease

## 7. Proliferative diabetic retinopathy

- Affects 5–10% of diabetics
- IDD at increased risk (60% after 30 years)

### Neovascularization

- Flat or elevated
- Severity determined by comparing with area of disc

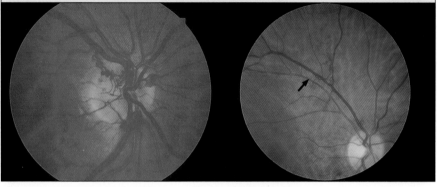

- Neovascularization of disc
- Neovascularization elsewhere

### Indications for treatment

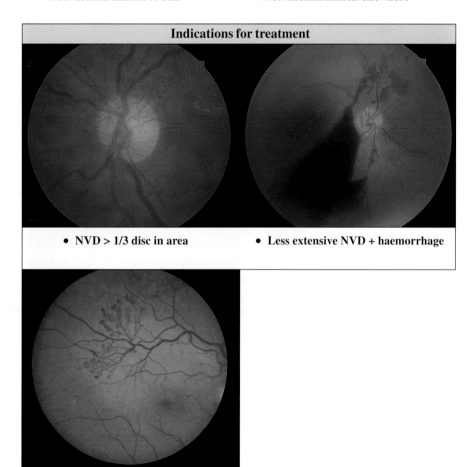

- NVD > 1/3 disc in area
- Less extensive NVD + haemorrhage

- NVE > 1/2 disc in area + haemorrhage

## Laser panretinal photocoagulation

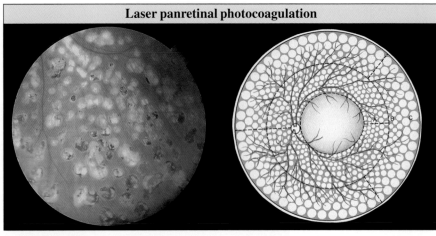

- Initial treatment is 2000–3000 burns
- Spot size (200–500 μm) depends on contact lens magnification
- Gentle intensity burn (0.10–0.05 sec)

- Area covered by complete PRP
- Follow-up 4–8 weeks

## Assessment after photocoagulation

| Poor involution | Good involution |
|---|---|

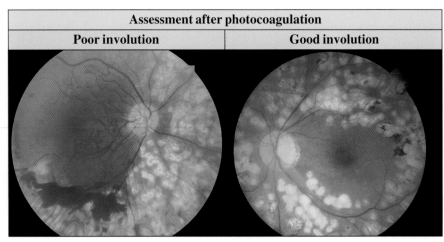

- Persistent neovascularization
- Haemorrhage
- Re-treatment required

- Regression of neovascularization
- Residual 'ghost' vessels or fibrous tissue
- Disc pallor

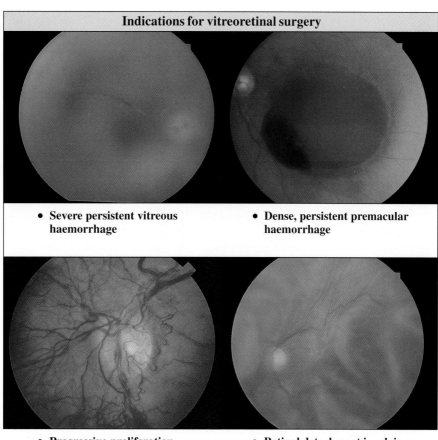

**Indications for vitreoretinal surgery**

- Severe persistent vitreous haemorrhage

- Dense, persistent premacular haemorrhage

- Progressive proliferation despite laser therapy

- Retinal detachment involving macula

# OTHER RETINAL VASCULAR DISORDERS

1. **Retinal vein occlusion**
   - Branch retinal vein occlusion
   - Central retinal vein occlusion

2. **Retinal artery occlusion**
   - Branch retinal artery occlusion
   - Cilioretinal artery occlusion
   - Central retinal artery occlusion

3. **Hypertensive retinopathy**

4. **Sickle-cell retinopathy**

5. **Retinopathy of prematurity**

6. **Retinal telangiectasias**
   - Idiopathic juxtafoveolar
   - Leber miliary aneurysms
   - Coats disease

7. **Retinal artery macroaneurysm**

8. **Retinopathy in blood dyscrasias**

9. **Radiation retinopathy**

## 1. Retinal vein occlusion

**PREDISPOSING FACTORS**

1. **Systemic**
   - **Increasing age**
   - **Hypertension**
   - **Diabetes**
   - **Abnormalities of coagulation**
2. **Ocular**
   - **Raised intraocular pressure**
   - **Periphlebitis**

**Pathophysiology**

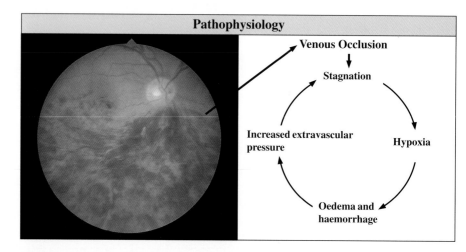

Venous Occlusion → Stagnation → Hypoxia → Oedema and haemorrhage → Increased extravascular pressure → Stagnation

## Branch retinal vein occlusion (BRVO)

**Signs of acute BRVO**

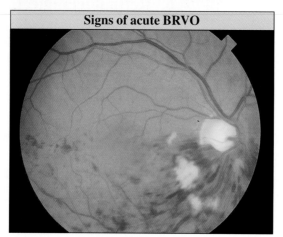

- **Venous tortuosity and dilatation**
- **Flame-shaped and 'dot-blot' haemorrhages**
- **Cotton-wool spots and retinal oedema**

*Prognosis*
- **VA 6/12 or better after 6 months in 50%**

*Complications*
- **Chronic macular oedema and neovascularization**

## Fluorescein angiogram

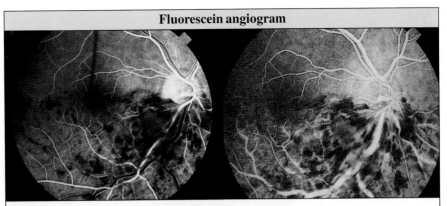

- Early – blocked background fluorescence due to haemorrhage

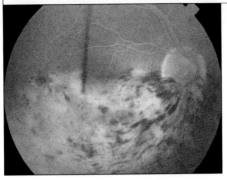

- Late – hyperfluorescence due to diffuse oedema

## Signs of old BRVO

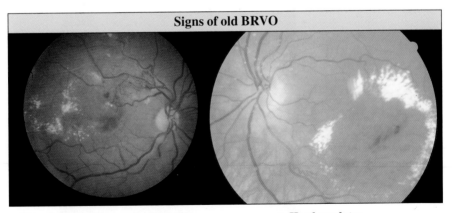

- Vascular sheathing and collaterals

- Hard exudates

## Management of chronic macular oedema

- Most common cause of persistent poor VA
- Wait 6–12 weeks and perform FA

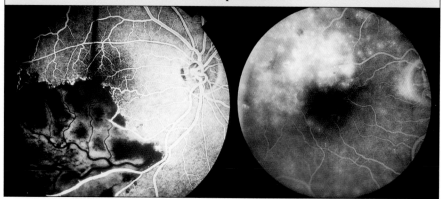

- Macular non-perfusion – no treatment
- Good macular perfusion and VA 6/18 or worse after 3 months – consider laser photocoagulation

## Management of neovascularization

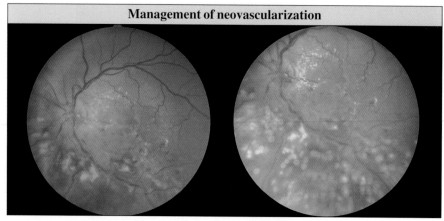

- Occurs in about 30–50% of eyes
- Most frequently after 6–12 months
- Perform laser photocoagulation to involved segment

**Central retinal vein occlusion (CRVO)**

## Signs of non-ischaemic CRVO

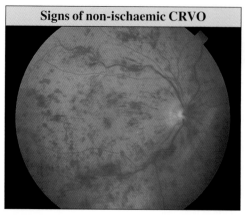

- VA > CF
- APD – mild
- Mild venous tortuosity and dilatation
- Mild to moderate retinal haemorrhages
- Variable cotton-wool spots
- Mild to moderate disc oedema
- Chronic macular oedema
- Guarded prognosis
- May subsequently convert to ischaemic

## Fluorescein angiogram of non-ischaemic CRVO

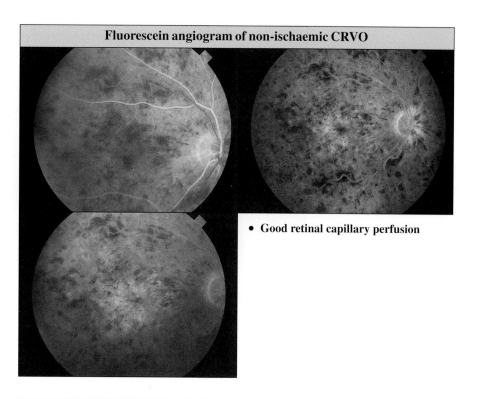

- Good retinal capillary perfusion

## Signs of ischaemic CRVO

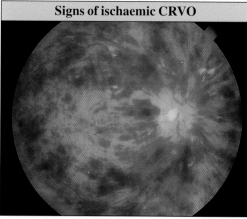

- VA < 6/60
- APD – marked
- Marked venous tortuosity and engorgement
- Extensive retinal haemorrhages
- Variable cotton-wool spots
- Severe disc oedema
- Macular ischaemia
- Very poor prognosis
- Rubeosis irides in 50%

## Fluorescein angiogram of ischaemic CRVO

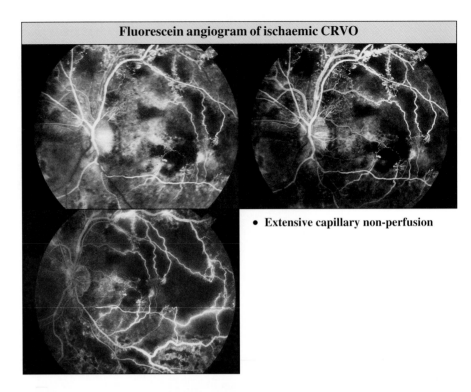

- Extensive capillary non-perfusion

## Management of ischaemic CRVO

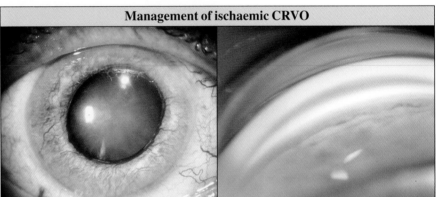

- Check every month for 6 months
- Look for rubeosis and angle new vessels

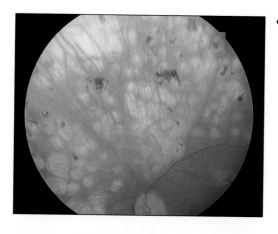

- Treat neovascularization by panretinal photocoagulation

| Papillophlebitis |
| --- |
| ● Affects healthy patients < 50 years |

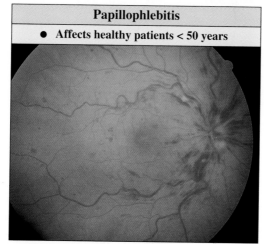

- VA – slight decrease
- APD – absent
- Venous tortuosity and dilatation
- Variable cotton-wool spots and haemorrhages
- Severe disc oedema
- Very good prognosis in 80%

2. Retinal artery occlusion

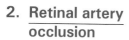

| Causes |
| --- |

Embolism

Vaso-obliteration

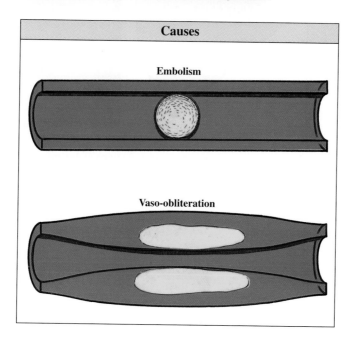

| Types of emboli | |
|---|---|
| **Cardiac** | **Carotid** |

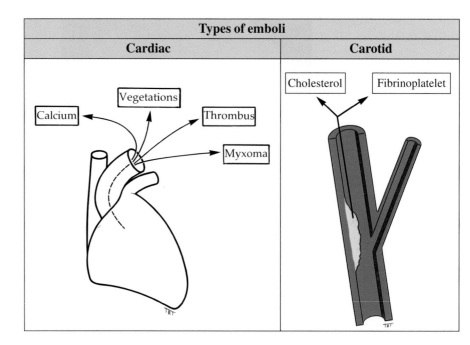

## Cholesterol emboli (Hollenhorst plaques)

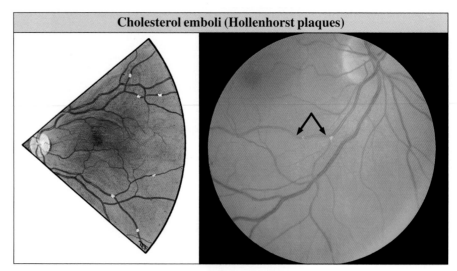

- Multiple, bright, refractile crystals
- Often located at arteriolar bifurcations
- Frequently asymptomatic

## Fibrinoplatelet emboli

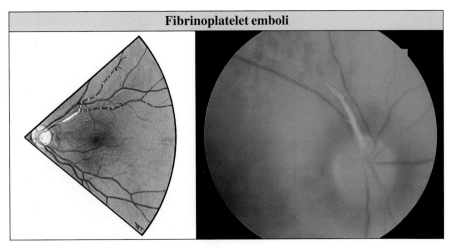

- Multiple, dull grey particles
- Occasionally fill entire lumen
- May cause amaurosis fugax and occasionally permanent obstruction

## Calcific emboli

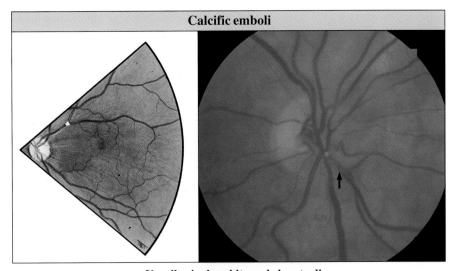

- Usually single, white and close to disc
- May cause permanent obstruction

| Causes of vaso-obliteration | |
|---|---|
| **Atherosclerosis** | **Periarteritis** |

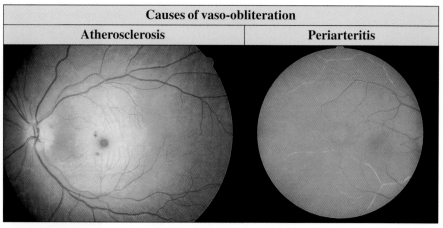

- Most common cause of central artery occlusion
- PAN and SLE may cause branch artery occlusion

- Haematological disorders may cause recurrent occlusions in young individuals
  - Protein S deficiency, protein C deficiency
  - Antithrombin III deficiency
  - 'Sticky platelet syndromes' and antiphospholipid antibody syndrome

**Branch retinal artery occlusion (BRAO)**

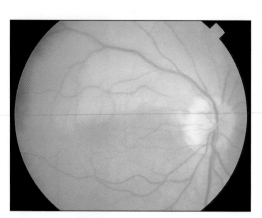

- VA – variable
- APD – mild or absent
- Retinal whitening
- Arteriolar narrowing

| Fluorescein angiogram of BRAO |
|---|

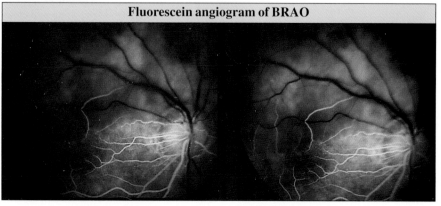

- Early masking
- Extreme delay of arterial phase

**Cilioretinal artery occlusion**

- Cilioretinal artery derived from posterior ciliary circulation
- Present in about 30% of individuals

| Isolated | Combined with CRVO |
|---|---|
| 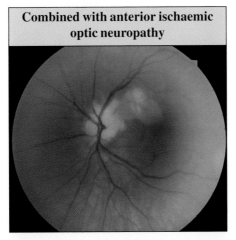 | |

- In young individuals with a systemic vasculitis
- Usually good prognosis

- Guarded prognosis

**Combined with anterior ischaemic optic neuropathy**

- Elderly patients with giant cell arteritis
- Very poor prognosis

**Central retinal artery occlusion (CRAO)**

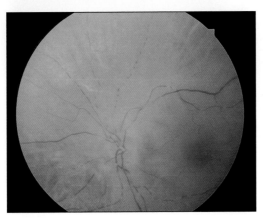

- VA < 6/60
- APD – marked
- Retinal whitening
- 'Cherry-red spot' at macula
- Arteriolar and venular narrowing
- Sludging and segmentation of blood column (cattle-trucking)
- Very poor prognosis

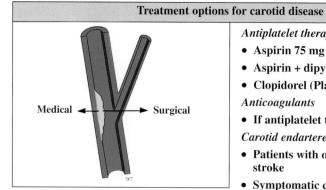

**Treatment options for carotid disease**

Medical ←→ Surgical

*Antiplatelet therapy*
- Aspirin 75 mg daily
- Aspirin + dipyridamole (Persantin)
- Clopidorel (Plavix) 75 mg daily

*Anticoagulants*
- If antiplatelet therapy ineffective

*Carotid endarterectomy*
- Patients with other risk factors for stroke
- Symptomatic carotid stenosis > 70%

## 3. Hypertensive retinopathy

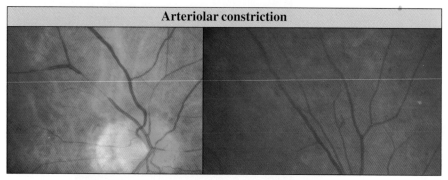

**Arteriolar constriction**

- Focal
- Generalized

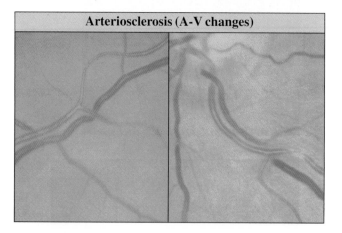

**Arteriosclerosis (A-V changes)**

## Extravascular signs

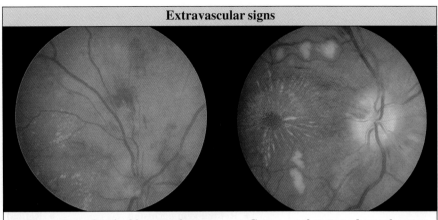

- Flame-shaped retinal haemorrhages
- Cotton-wool spots and macular star

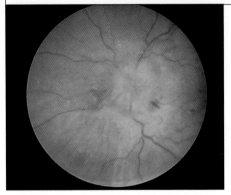

- Disc oedema

## Grading of arteriosclerosis

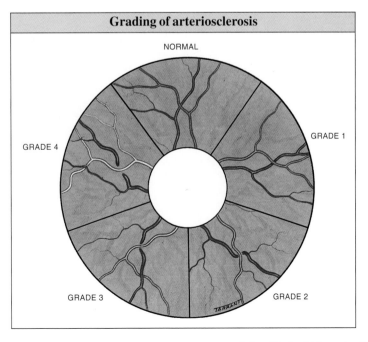

NORMAL

GRADE 1

GRADE 2

GRADE 3

GRADE 4

## Ocular associations

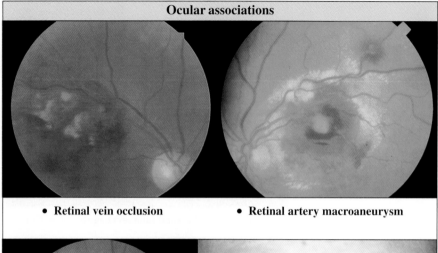

- Retinal vein occlusion
- Retinal artery macroaneurysm

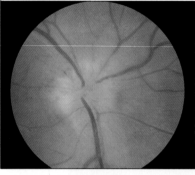 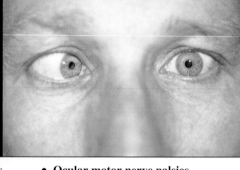

- Anterior ischaemic optic neuropathy
- Ocular motor nerve palsies

### 4. Sickle-cell retinopathy

## Staging of proliferative

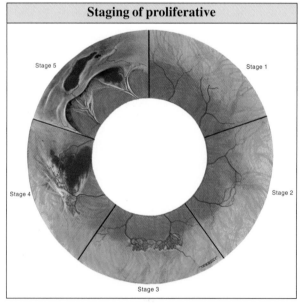

Stage 5    Stage 1

Stage 4    Stage 2

Stage 3

- Peripheral arteriolar occlusion (1)
- Peripheral arteriovenous anastomoses (2)
- Neovascularization ('sea-fan') (3)
- Vitreous haemorrhage (4)
- Fibrovascular proliferation and traction (5)

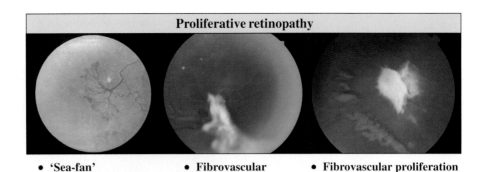

**Proliferative retinopathy**

- 'Sea-fan' neovascularization
- Fibrovascular proliferation
- Fibrovascular proliferation and bleeding

**Non-proliferative retinopathy**

- Salmon patches (equatorial haemorrhages)
- Black sunbursts (RPE hyperplasia)
- Retinal holes

## 5. Retinopathy of pre-maturity (ROP)

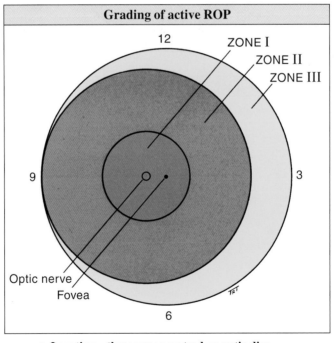

**Grading of active ROP**

- Location – three zones centred on optic disc
- Extent – number of clock hours involved

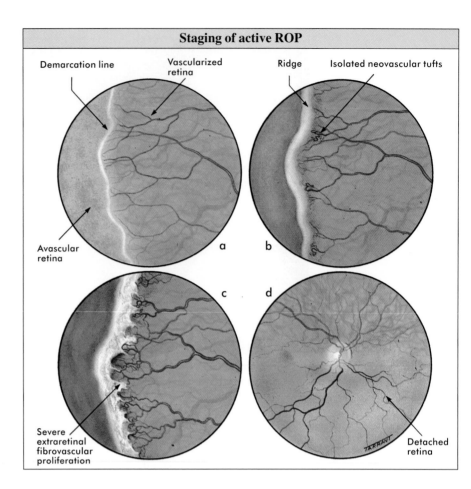

**Staging of active ROP**

Demarcation line

Vascularized retina

Ridge

Isolated neovascular tufts

Avascular retina

a

b

c

d

Severe extraretinal fibrovascular proliferation

Detached retina

## TREATMENT OF ACTIVE ROP

1. **Modality**
   - **Cryotherapy**
   - **Laser photocoagulation**
2. **Indications – threshold disease**
   **(5 contiguous or 8 non-contiguous clock hours in zone I or zone II, associated with 'plus' disease)**
3. **Results**
   - **75% success**
   - **25% progress to detachment despite treatment**

## Cicatricial ROP

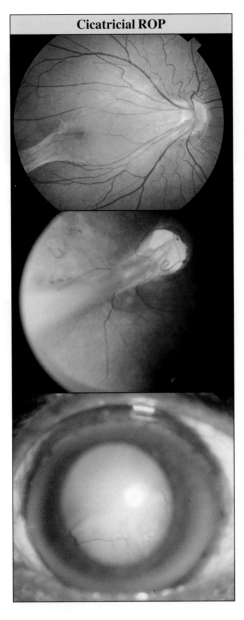

- Temporal vitreoretinal fibrosis and dragging of disc

- Falciform retinal fold

- Total retinal detachment

## 6. Retinal telangiectasias

**Idiopathic juxtafoveolar**

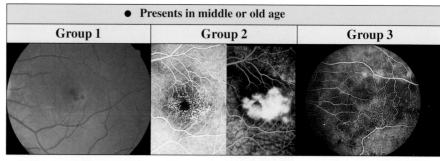

| | Presents in middle or old age | |
|---|---|---|
| **Group 1** | **Group 2** | **Group 3** |
| • Unilateral, telangiectasia temporal to fovea<br>• May benefit from photocoagulation<br>• Good prognosis | • Bilateral, symmetrical perifoveal telangiectasia<br>• Occasionally may benefit from photocoagulation<br>• Guarded prognosis | • Bilateral, severe, perifoveal telangiectasia and capillary occlusion<br>• Photocoagulation not beneficial<br>• Poor prognosis |

**Leber miliary aneurysms**

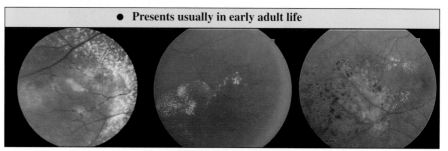

● Presents usually in early adult life

- Temporal fusiform and saccular vascular dilatation
- Hard exudates may threaten macula
- Photocoagulation may be beneficial

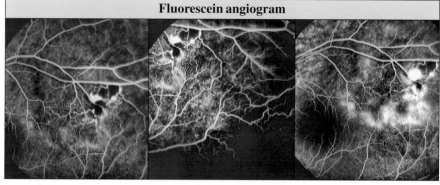

**Fluorescein angiogram**

- Localized dilatation
- Associated non-perfusion
- Leakage

**Coats disease**

| Presentation |
|---|

- First decade, more common in boys
- Always unilateral

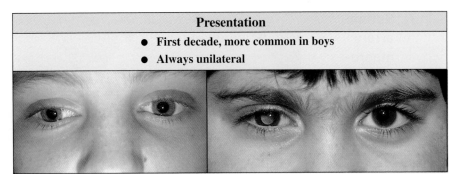

- Visual loss and strabismus
- White fundus reflex (leukocoria)

| Progression |
|---|

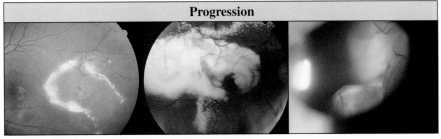

- Retinal and subretinal hard exudation
- Overlying vascular dilatation and tortuosity
- May benefit from photocoagulation

- Slow progresssion of exudation
- Severe visual loss
- Treatment not beneficial

- Exudative retinal detachment and retrolental mass
- May mimic retinoblastoma

| Fluorescein angiogram |
|---|

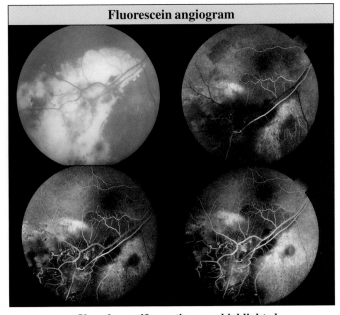

- Vascular malformations are highlighted

## 7. Retinal artery macro-aneurysm

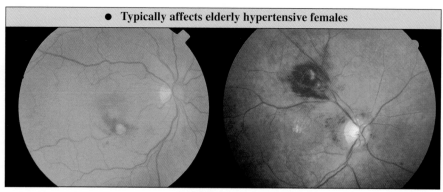

● Typically affects elderly hypertensive females

● Localized dilatation of retinal arteriole

● Most frequently along temporal arcades

● Surrounding retinal haemorrhage

● Spontaneous involution is common

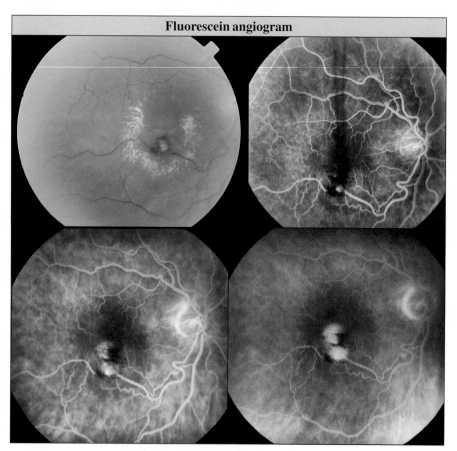

**Fluorescein angiogram**

● Immediate uniform filling of macroaneurysm

● Late leakage

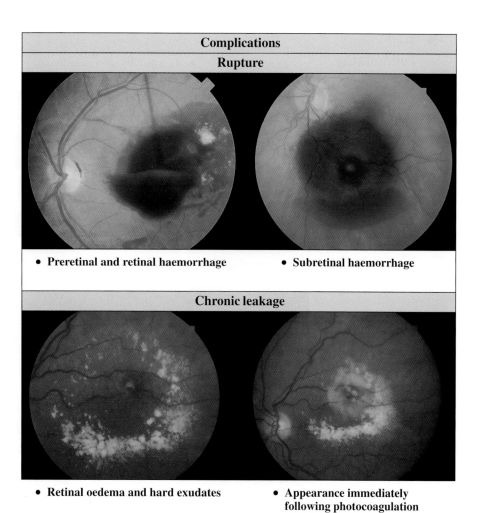

| Complications | |
|---|---|
| **Rupture** | |

- Preretinal and retinal haemorrhage
- Subretinal haemorrhage

| **Chronic leakage** | |
|---|---|

- Retinal oedema and hard exudates
- Appearance immediately following photocoagulation

## 8. Retinopathy in blood dyscrasias

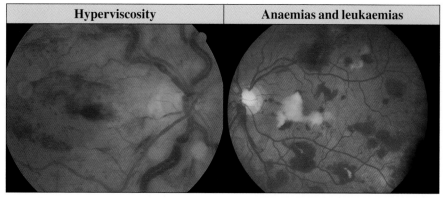

| Hyperviscosity | Anaemias and leukaemias |
|---|---|

- Venous dilatation, segmentation and tortuosity
- Haemorrhages

- Haemorrhages, cotton-wool spots and venous tortuosity
- Occasionally Roth spots

## 9. Radiation retinopathy

- Latent interval 6 months to 3 years

- Hard exudates and small flame-shaped haemorrhages

- Increase in hard exudate formation

- Arteriolar occlusion, cotton-wool spots and haemorrhages

- Proliferative retinopathy, vitreous haemorrhage and retinal detachment

# CHILDHOOD STRABISMUS

1. **Examination**

2. **Esotropia**
   - Essential infantile esotropia
   - Refractive accommodative esotropia
   - Non-refractive accommodative esotropia

3. **Exotropia**
   - Constant exotropia
   - Intermittent exotropia

4. **Special syndromes**
   - Duane syndrome
   - Brown syndrome
   - Double elevator palsy
   - Möbius syndrome

5. **Alphabet patterns**
   - 'V' pattern deviation
   - 'A' pattern deviation

## 1. Examination

**Visual acuity tests in preverbal children**

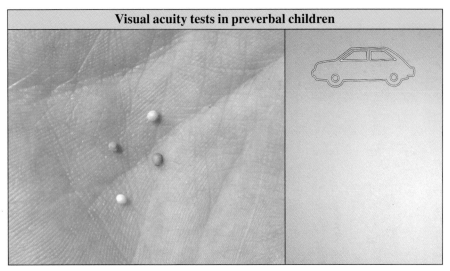

- 'Hundreds and thousands' sweet test
- Preferential looking with Cardiff cards

**Visual acuity tests in verbal children**

**At age 2 years (naming pictures)**

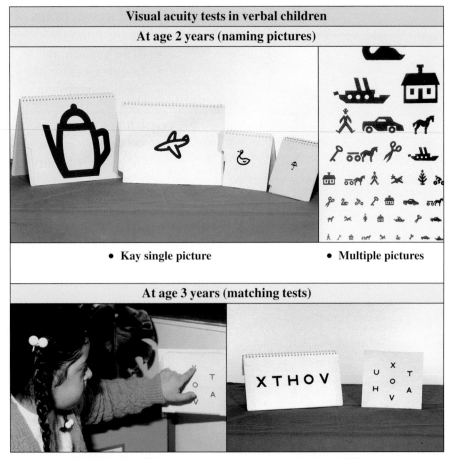

- Kay single picture
- Multiple pictures

**At age 3 years (matching tests)**

- Sheridan–Gardiner
- Sonksen–Silver

## Tests for stereopsis

### Titmus

- Polaroid spectacles
- Figures seen in 3-D

### TNO random dot test

- Red-green spectacles
- 'Hidden' shapes seen

### Frisby

- No spectacles
- 'Hidden' circle seen

## Lang

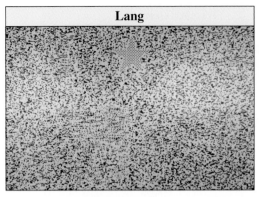

- No spectacles
- Shapes seen

## Tests for sensory anomalies

| Worth four-dot test | Bagolini striated glasses |
|---|---|

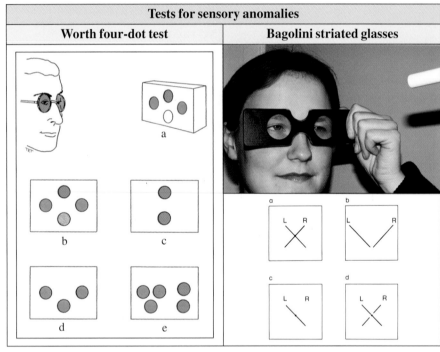

- Prior to use of glasses (a)
- Normal or ARC (b)
- Left suppression (c)
- Right suppression (d)
- Diplopia (e)

- Normal or ARC (a)
- Diplopia (b)
- Suppression (c)
- Small suppression scotoma (d)

## Synoptophore

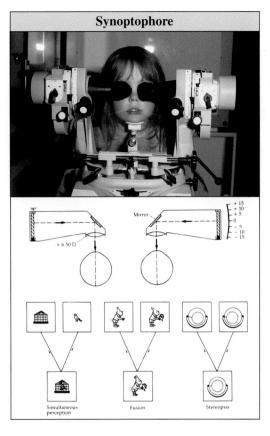

- Grading of binocular vision
- Detection of suppression and ARC
- Measurement of angle
- Measurement of fusional amplitudes

Simultaneous perception    Fusion    Stereopsis

## Dissimilar image tests

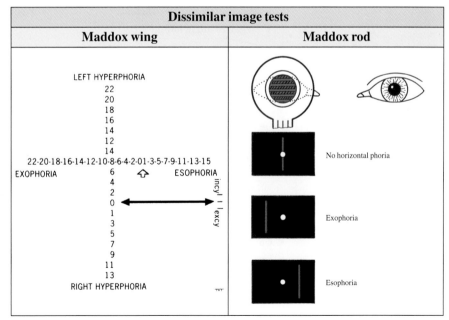

| Maddox wing | Maddox rod |
|---|---|
| LEFT HYPERPHORIA<br>22<br>20<br>18<br>16<br>14<br>12<br>14<br>22-20-18-16-14-12-10-8-6-4-2-01-3-5-7-9-11-13-15<br>EXOPHORIA   6   ⇧   ESOPHORIA<br>4<br>2<br>0   incyl ⟷ excy<br>1<br>3<br>5<br>7<br>9<br>11<br>13<br>RIGHT HYPERPHORIA | No horizontal phoria<br><br>Exophoria<br><br>Esophoria |

- Dissociates eyes for near fixation (1/3 m)
- Measures heterophoria

- White spot converted into red streak
- Cannot differentiate tropia from phoria

### Hirschberg test

- Rough measure of deviation
- Note location of corneal light reflex
- 1 mm = 7° or 15 △

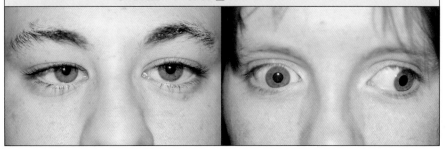

- Reflex at border of pupil = 15 △
- Reflex at limbus = 45 △

### Pseudo-deviations

| Pseudo-esotropia | Pseudo-exotropia |
| --- | --- |

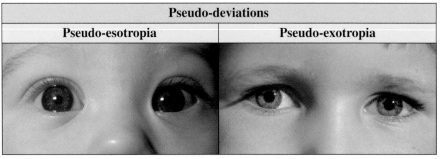

- Epicanthic folds
- Short interpupillary distance
- Negative angle kappa

- Wide interpupillary distance
- Positive angle kappa

### Cover tests

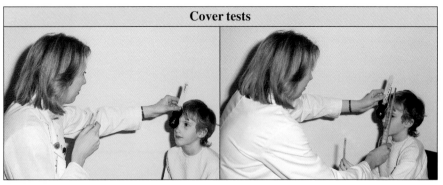

- Cover test detects heterotropia
- Uncover test detects heterophoria
- Alternate cover test detects total deviation

- Prism cover test measures total deviation

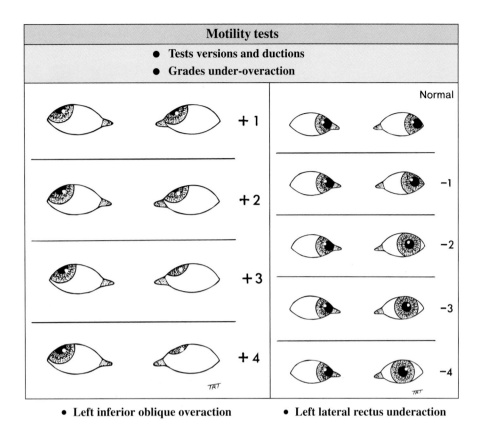

**Motility tests**

- **Tests versions and ductions**
- **Grades under-overaction**

Normal

+ 1

+ 2

+ 3

+ 4

−1

−2

−3

−4

- **Left inferior oblique overaction**
- **Left lateral rectus underaction**

## 2. Esotropia

**Essential infantile esotropia**

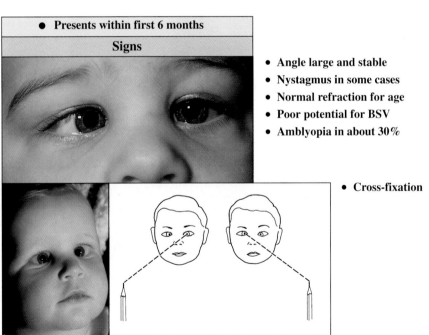

- **Presents within first 6 months**

**Signs**

- Angle large and stable
- Nystagmus in some cases
- Normal refraction for age
- Poor potential for BSV
- Amblyopia in about 30%

- **Cross-fixation**

| Management |
|---|

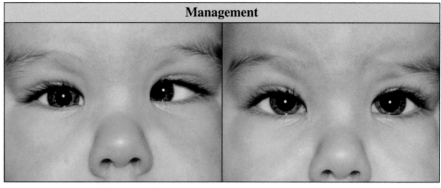

- Correct amblyopia if present
- Surgery before age 18 months

- Bilateral medial rectus recessions
- Ideal alignment within 10 △

| Subsequent problems |
|---|
| **Inferior oblique overaction** |

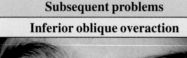

- Most common onset 2 years
- Usually eventually bilateral

| **Dissociated vertical deviation** |
|---|

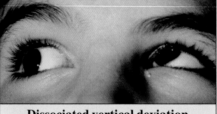

- Up-drift with excyclodeviation of eye under cover
- When cover removed affected eye moves down

| **Microtropia** |
|---|

- Very small angle – may not be detectable on cover testing
- Central suppression scotoma

**Refractive accommodative esotropia**

- Presents between 18 months and 3 years
- Initially intermittent
- Normal AC/A ratio
- Excessive hypermetropia

| Fully accommodative | Partially accommodative |
|---|---|

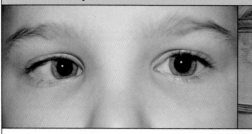 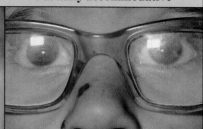

- Esotropia greater for near
- Straight for distance

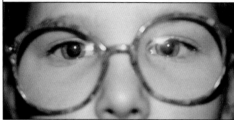 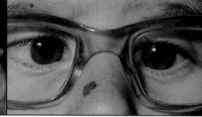

- Straight for distance and near
- Esotropia for near

**Non-refractive accommodative esotropia**

- Presents between 18 months and 3 years
- High AC/A ratio
  - due to increased AC (convergence excess)
  - due to decreased A (hypoaccommodative)
- No significant refractive error

**Signs**

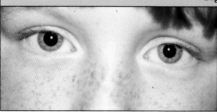 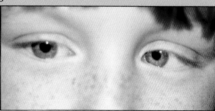

- Straight for distance
- Esotropia for near

| Management |
| --- |
| • **Refraction – prescribe full cycloplegic refraction under age 6 years** |
| **Treatment of amblyopia** |

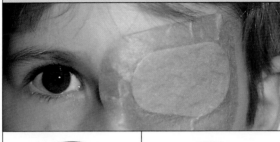

Surgery – if spectacles do not fully correct deviation

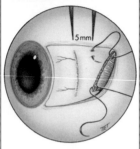

• **Recession**

• **Resection**

## 3. Exotropia

**Constant exotropia**

| Congenital | Sensory |
| --- | --- |

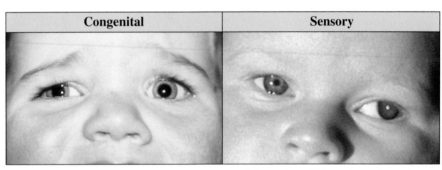

- • Presents at birth
- • Large angle
- • Alternating fixation
- • Normal refraction for age

- • Disruption of binocular reflexes by acquired lesions, such as cataract

*Consecutive*
- • Follows previous surgery for esotropia

**Intermittent exotropia**

| Signs |
|---|
| 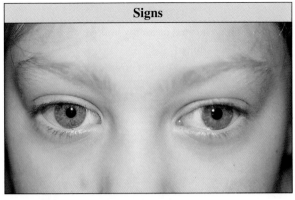 |

*Basic*
- Angle greater for near

*Convergence weakness*
- Angle greater for near
- May be associated with myopia

*Divergence excess*
- Angle greater for distance
- May be true or simulated

- Presents – usually prior to 5 years
- Usually alternating (amblyopia uncommon)
- Treatment – surgery

## 4. Special syndromes

**Duane syndrome**

- Bilateral in about 20%
- On attempted adduction–retraction of globe and narrowing of palpebral fissure
- On attempted abduction–opening of palpebral fissure and normal globe position

| Type I (left) |
|---|
| 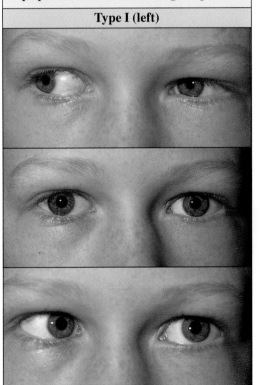 |

- Adduction – normal or mildly limited

- Primary position – straight or mild esotropia

- Abduction – limited or absent

| Type II |
|---|
| • Abduction – normal or mildly limited |
| • Adduction – limited |
| • Primary position – straight or mild exotropia |
| **Type III (left)** |

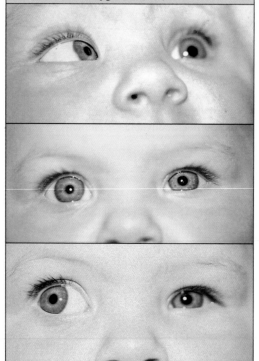

• Abduction – limited

• Primary position – straight or mild esotropia

• Adduction – limited

**Brown syndrome**

| Brown syndrome (right) |
|---|

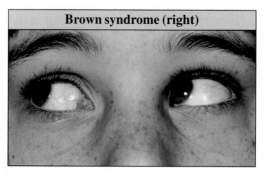

• Normal elevation in abduction

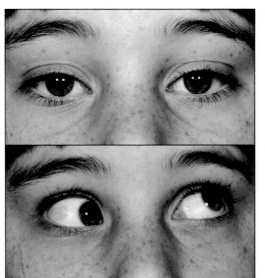

- Straight in primary position

- Limited elevation in adduction

**Double elevator palsy**

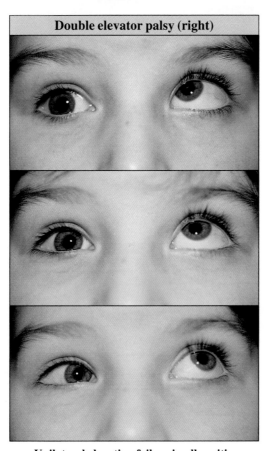

Double elevator palsy (right)

- Unilateral elevation failure in all positions

**Möbius syndrome**

| Signs |
|---|
| 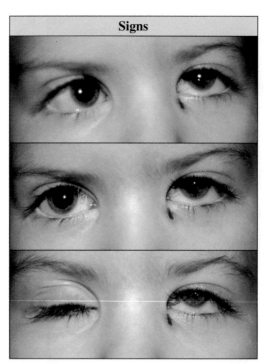 |

- Bilateral sixth nerve palsies – patient looking left

- Primary position – 50% straight, 50% esotropic
- Horizontal gaze palsy in 50%

- Bilateral, usually asymmetrical facial palsies sparing lower face
- Paresis of 9th and 12th cranial nerves

## 5. Alphabet patterns

### 'V' pattern deviation

| Signs | Treatment |
|---|---|
| 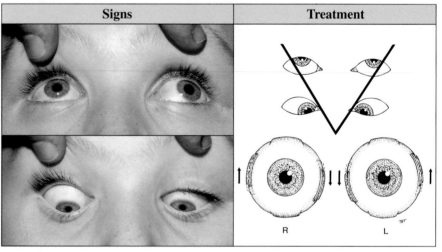 | |

- Difference between up- and downgaze is 15 △ or more

*'V' pattern esotropia*
- Bilateral medial rectus recessions + downward transposition

*'V' pattern exotropia*
- Bilateral lateral rectus recessions + upward transpositions

**'A' pattern deviation**

| Signs | Treatment |
|---|---|
| 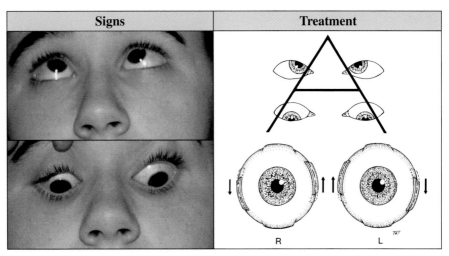 | |

- Difference between up- and downgaze 10 △ or more

*'A' pattern esotropia*
- Bilateral medial rectus recessions + upward transposition

*'A' pattern exotropia*
- Bilateral lateral rectus recessions + downward transposition

# THYROID EYE DISEASE

1. Soft tissue involvement

2. Eyelid retraction

3. Proptosis

4. Optic neuropathy

5. Restrictive myopathy

**1. Soft tissue involvement**

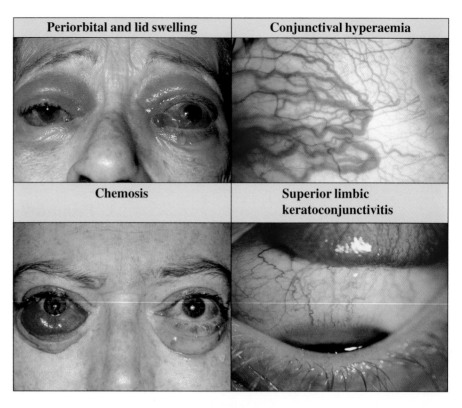

| Periorbital and lid swelling | Conjunctival hyperaemia |
| --- | --- |
| Chemosis | Superior limbic keratoconjunctivitis |

**2. Eyelid retraction**

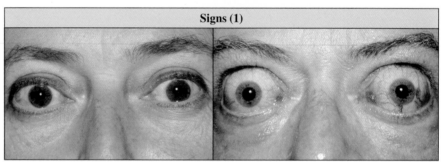

Signs (1)

- Bilateral lid retraction
- No associated proptosis

- Bilateral lid retraction
- Bilateral proptosis

| Signs (2) |
|---|

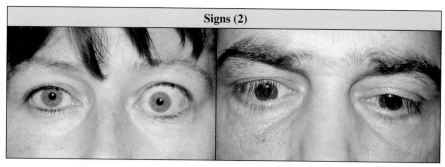

- Unilateral lid retraction
- Unilateral proptosis

- Lid lag in downgaze

## 3. Proptosis

- Occurs in about 50%
- Uninfluenced by treatment of hyperthyroidism

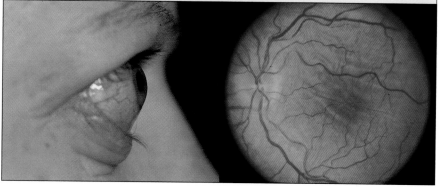

- Axial and permanent in about 70%
- May be associated with choroidal folds

*Treatment options*

- Systemic steroids
- Radiotherapy
- Surgical decompression

## 4. Optic neuropathy

- Occurs in about 5%
- Early defective colour vision
- Usually normal disc appearance

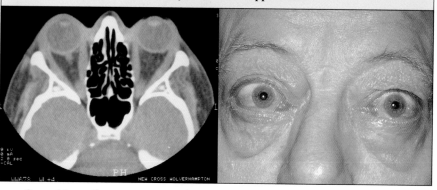

- Caused by optic nerve compression at orbital apex by enlarged recti
- Often occurs in absence of significant proptosis

## 5. Restrictive myopathy

- Occurs in about 40%
- Due to fibrotic contracture

### Signs

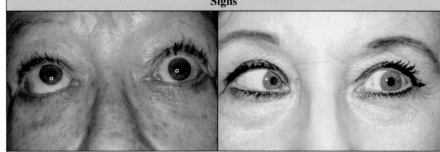

- Elevation defect – most common
- Abduction defect – less common

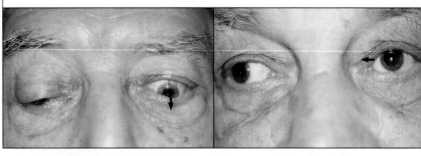

- Depression defect – uncommon
- Adduction defect – rare

# ORBITAL INFECTIONS AND INFLAMMATIONS

1.  **Orbital cellulitis**

2.  **Idiopathic orbital inflammatory disease**

3.  **Dacryoadenitis**

4.  **Orbital myositis**

## 1. Orbital cellulitis

- Infection behind orbital septum
- Usually secondary to ethmoiditis
- Presents – severe malaise, fever and orbital signs

### Signs

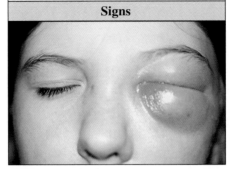

- Severe eyelid oedema and redness
- Proptosis – most frequently lateral and down
- Painful ophthalmoplegia
- Optic nerve dysfunction if advanced

### Complications

- Raised intraocular pressure
- Retinal vascular occlusion
- Optic neuropathy

| Orbital | Intracranial |
|---|---|

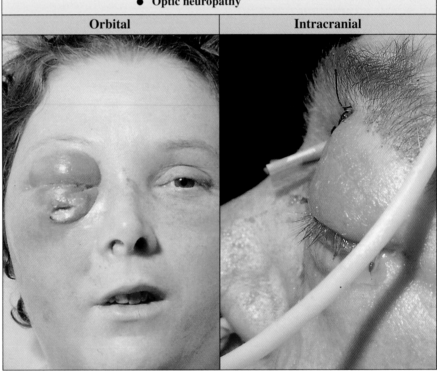

| Orbital | Intracranial |
|---|---|
| • Orbital or subperiosteal abscess | • Meningitis, brain abscess<br>• Cavernous sinus thrombosis |

## Management

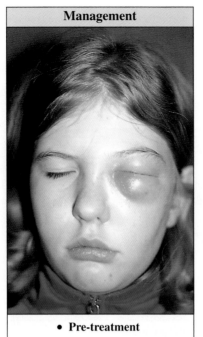

- Pre-treatment

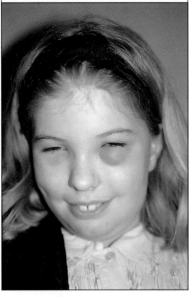

- Post-treatment

1. Hospital admission

2. Systemic antibiotic therapy

3. Monitoring of optic nerve function

4. Indications for surgery
   - Resistance to antibodies
   - Orbital or subperiosteal abscess
   - Optic neuropathy

## 2. Idiopathic orbital inflammatory disease (IOID)

- Non-neoplastic, non-infectious orbital lesion (pseudotumour)
- Involves any or all soft-tissue components
- Presents – 20–50 years with abrupt painful onset

### Signs

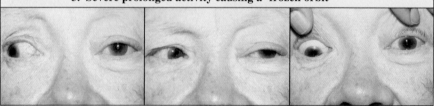

- Usually unilateral
- Periorbital swelling and chemosis
- Proptosis
- Ophthalmoplegia

### Clinical course and treatment

**1. Early spontaneous remission without sequelae**

*Treatment*
- Nil

**2. Prolonged intermittent activity with eventual remission**

*Treatment options*
- Steroids
- Radiotherapy or
- Cytotoxics

**3. Severe prolonged activity causing a 'frozen orbit'**

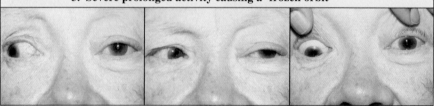

- Left involvement resulting in ophthalmoplegia and ptosis

**3. Dacryo-adenitis**

- Usually affects otherwise healthy individuals – no treatment required
- Presents – acute discomfort over lacrimal gland

**Signs**

- Oedema of lateral aspect of upper lid
- Mild downward and inward globe displacement
- Injection and tenderness of palpebral lobe of lacrimal gland
- Reduction in tear secretion

**4. Orbital myositis**

- Subtype of IOID
- Involvement of one or more extraocular muscles
- Clinical course is usually short
- Presents – sudden onset of pain on ocular movement

**Signs**

- Underaction of left lateral rectus
- Worsening of pain on attempted left gaze
- CT shows fusiform enlargement of left lateral rectus

# VASCULAR ORBITAL DISORDERS

1. **Orbital venous anomalies (varices)**
   - Isolated orbital varices
   - Combined orbital and external varices

2. **Carotid-cavernous fistula**
   - Direct
   - Indirect (dural shunt)

## 1. Orbital venous anomalies (varices)

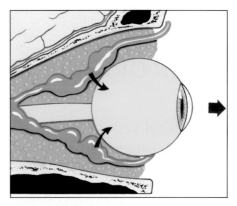

- Congenital enlargements of pre-existing venous channels
- Usually unilateral
- May bleed or become thrombosed

**Isolated orbital varices**

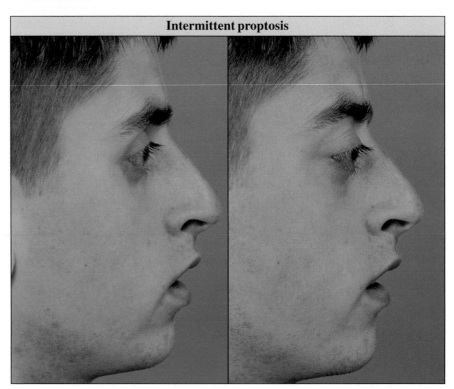

**Intermittent proptosis**

- Non-pulsatile, without a bruit
- Precipitated or accentuated by Valsalva manoeuvre

**Combined orbital and external varices**

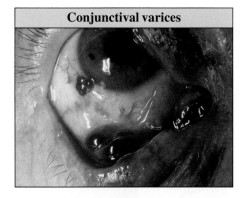

**Conjunctival varices**

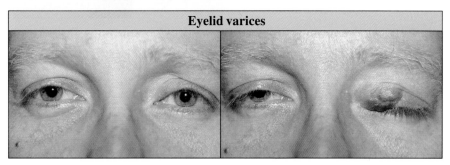

**Eyelid varices**

- Precipitated or accentuated by Valsalva manoeuvre

## 2. Carotid-cavernous fistula

**Direct**

- Defect in intracavernous part of internal carotid
- Rapid-flow shunt

*Causes*

- Head trauma – most common
- Spontaneous rupture – in hypertensive females

**Signs (1)**

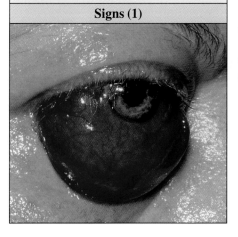

- Ptosis, chemosis and conjunctival injection
- Ophthalmoplegia
- Raised intraocular pressure

## Signs (2)

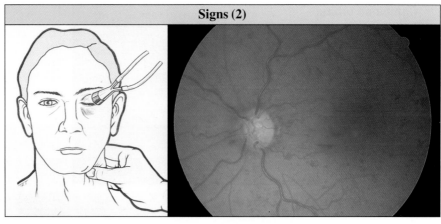

- Pulsatile proptosis with bruit and thrill
- Abolished by ipsilateral carotid compression

- Retinal venous congestion and haemorrhages

**Indirect (dural shunt)**

- Indirect communication between meningeal branches of internal or external carotids and cavernous sinus
- Slow-flow shunt

*Causes*

- Congenital malformations
- Spontaneous rupture

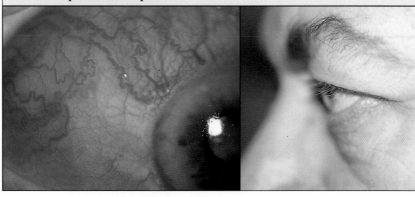

- Dilated episcleral vessels
- Raised intraocular pressure with wide pulsation

- Occasional ophthalmoplegia and mild proptosis

# ORBITAL TUMOURS

## 1. Vascular tumours
- Capillary haemangioma
- Cavernous haemangioma

## 2. Lacrimal gland tumours
- Pleomorphic adenoma
- Carcinoma

## 3. Neural tumours
- Optic nerve glioma
- Optic nerve sheath meningioma
- Sphenoidal ridge meningioma

## 4. Miscellaneous tumours
- Lymphoma
- Rhabdomyosarcoma
- Metastases
- Invasion from sinuses

## 1. Vascular tumours

### Capillary haemangioma

- Most common orbital tumour in children
- Presents – 30% at birth and 100% at 6 months

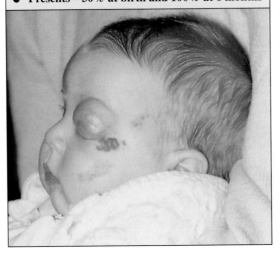

- Most commonly in superior anterior orbit
- May enlarge on coughing or straining
- Associated 'strawberry' naevus is common

**Natural history**

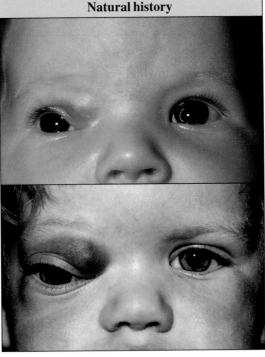

*Systemic associations*
- High output cardiac failure
- Kasabach–Merritt syndrome – thrombocytopenia, anaemia
- Maffuci syndrome – skin haemangiomas, enchondromata

- Growth during first year
- Subsequent resolution – complete in 70% by age 7 years

*Treatment*
- Steroid injections – for superficial component
- Systemic steroids
- Local resection – difficult

**Cavernous haemangioma**

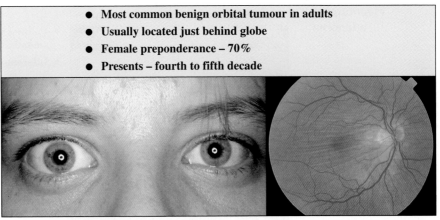

- Most common benign orbital tumour in adults
- Usually located just behind globe
- Female preponderance – 70%
- Presents – fourth to fifth decade

- Slowly progressive axial proptosis
- May cause choroidal folds

*Treatment*

- Surgical excision

## 2. Lacrimal gland tumours

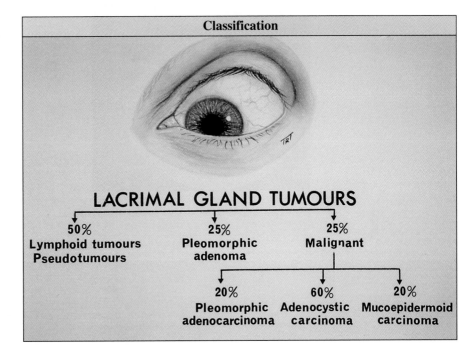

**Classification**

**LACRIMAL GLAND TUMOURS**

| 50% | 25% | 25% |
|---|---|---|
| Lymphoid tumours Pseudotumours | Pleomorphic adenoma | Malignant |

| 20% | 60% | 20% |
|---|---|---|
| Pleomorphic adenocarcinoma | Adenocystic carcinoma | Mucoepidermoid carcinoma |

**Pleomorphic adenoma**

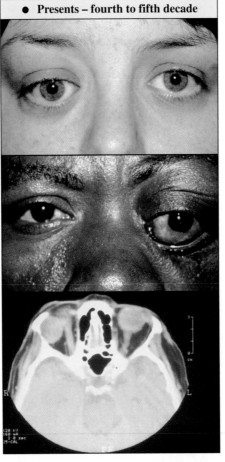

- Presents – fourth to fifth decade

- Painless and very slow-growing, smooth mass in lacrimal fossa
- Inferonasal globe displacement

- Posterior extension may cause proptosis and ophthalmoplegia

- Smooth, encapsulated outline
- Excavation of lacrimal gland fossa without destruction

| Technique of surgical excision | |
| --- | --- |
| ● Biopsy is contraindicated<br>● Prognosis – good if completely excised | |
| Incision of temporal muscle and periosteum | Drilling of bone for subsequent wiring |
| Removal of lateral orbital wall and dissection of tumour | Repair of temporal muscle and periosteum |

**Carcinoma**

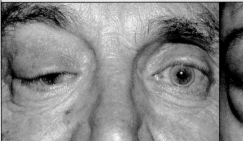
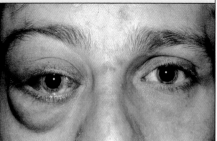

- Presents – fourth to sixth decades
- Very poor prognosis

- Painful, fast-growing mass in lacrimal fossa
- Inferonasal globe displacement

- Posterior extension may cause proptosis, ophthalmoplegia and episcleral congestion
- Trigeminal hypoaesthesia in 25%

*Treatment*
- Biopsy
- Radical surgery and radiotherapy

## 3. Neural tumours

### Optic nerve glioma

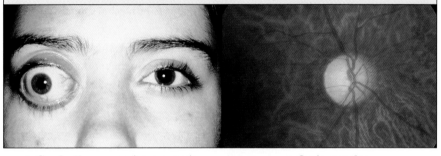

- Typically affects young girls
- Associated neurofibromatosis – 1 is common
- Presents – end of first decade with gradual visual loss

- Gradually progressive proptosis
- Optic atrophy

*Treatment*
- Observation – no growth, good vision and good cosmesis
- Excision – poor vision and poor cosmesis
- Radiotherapy – intracranial extension

**Optic nerve sheath meningioma**

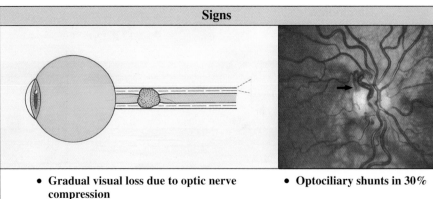

- Gradual visual loss due to optic nerve compression
- Optociliary shunts in 30%

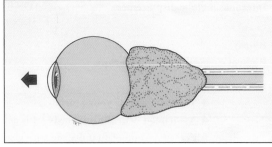
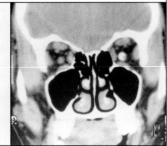

- Proptosis due to intraconal spread
- Thickening and calcification on CT

*Treatment*

- Observation – slow-growing tumours
- Excision – aggressive tumours and poor vision
- Radiotherapy – slow-growing tumours and good vision

**Sphenoidal ridge meningioma**

Signs

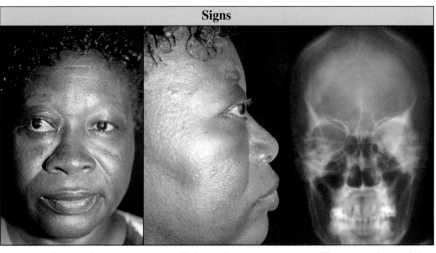

- Proptosis
- Fullness in temporal fossa
- Hyperostosis on plain X-ray

# 4. Miscellaneous tumours

## Lymphoma

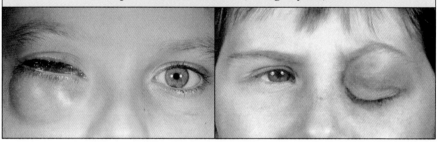

- Affects any part of orbit and may be bilateral
- Anterior lesions are rubbery on palpation
- May be confined to lacrimal glands

*Treatment*

- Radiotherapy – localized lesions
- Chemotherapy – disseminated disease

## Rhabdomyosarcoma

- Most common primary childhood orbital malignancy
- Rapid onset in first decade (average 7 years)

- May involve any part of orbit
- Palpable mass and ptosis in about 30%

*Treatment*

- Radiotherapy and chemotherapy
- Exenteration for radio-resistant or recurrent tumours

**Metastases**

| Childhood metastatic tumours | |
|---|---|
| **Neuroblastoma** | **Chloroma** |

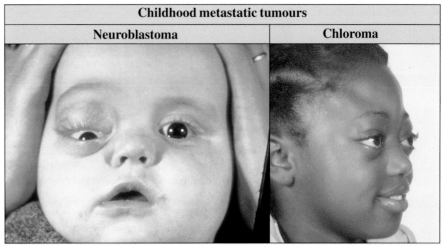

- Presents in early childhood
- May be bilateral
- Typically involves superior orbit

- Presents at about age 7 years
- Rapid onset proptosis – may be bilateral
- Subsequent systematic dissemination to full-blown leukaemia

**Adult metastatic tumours**

- Common primary sites – breast, bronchus, prostate, skin melanoma, gastrointestinal tract and kidney

**Presentations**

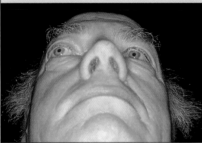 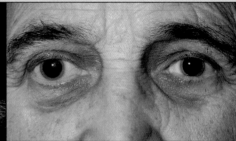

- Anterior orbital mass with non-axial globe displacement

- Enophthalmos with schirrous tumours

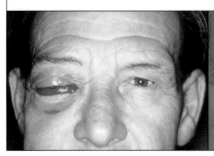

- Similar to orbital pseudotumour

- Cranial nerve involvement at orbital apex and mild proptosis

**Invasion from sinuses**

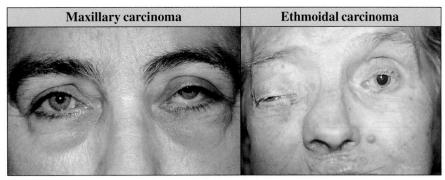

| Maxillary carcinoma | Ethmoidal carcinoma |

- Upward globe displacement and epiphora
- Lateral globe displacement

# OPTIC NEUROPATHIES

1. **Clinical features**

2. **Special investigations**

3. **Optic neuritis**
   - **Retrobulbar neuritis**
   - **Papillitis**
   - **Neuroretinitis**

4. **Anterior ischaemic optic neuropathy**
   - **Non-arteritic**
   - **Arteritic**

5. **Leber hereditary optic neuropathy**

## 1. Clinical features

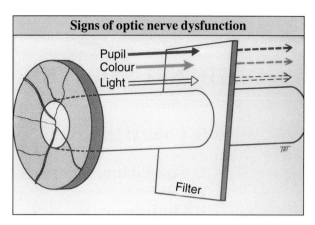

**Signs of optic nerve dysfunction**

- Pupil
- Colour
- Light
- Filter

- Reduced visual acuity
- Afferent pupillary conduction defect
- Dyschromatopsia
- Diminished light brightness sensitivity

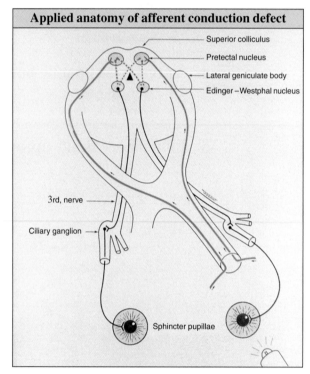

**Applied anatomy of afferent conduction defect**

- Superior colliculus
- Pretectal nucleus
- Lateral geniculate body
- Edinger–Westphal nucleus
- 3rd, nerve
- Ciliary ganglion
- Sphincter pupillae

*Signs*

- Equal pupil size
- Light reaction
  - ipsilateral direct is absent or diminished
  - consensual is normal
- Near reflex is normal in both eyes
- Total defect (no PL) = amaurotic pupil
- Relative defect = Marcus Gunn pupil

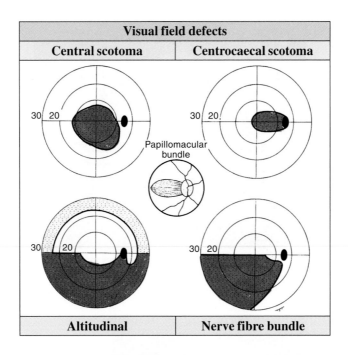

| Visual field defects | |
|---|---|
| Central scotoma | Centrocaecal scotoma |
| | *Papillomacular bundle* |
| Altitudinal | Nerve fibre bundle |

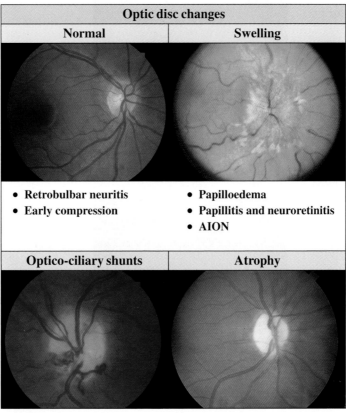

| Optic disc changes | |
|---|---|
| Normal | Swelling |
| • Retrobulbar neuritis<br>• Early compression | • Papilloedema<br>• Papillitis and neuroretinitis<br>• AION |
| Optico-ciliary shunts | Atrophy |
| • Optic nerve sheath meningioma<br>• Occasionally optic nerve glioma | • Postneuritic<br>• Compression<br>• Hereditary optic atrophies |

2. **Special investigations**

| MRI | Visually evoked potential |
|---|---|
| 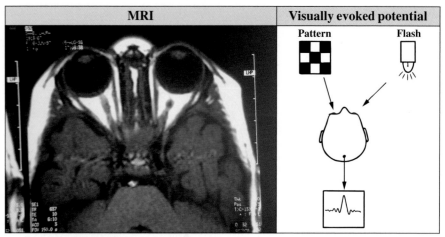 | |

Pattern      Flash

- Orbital fat-suppression techniques in T1-weighted images
- Assessment of electrical activity of visual cortex created by retinal stimulation

3. **Optic neuritis**

**Retrobulbar neuritis**

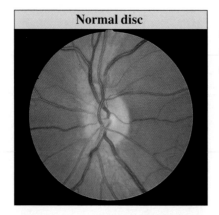

**Normal disc**

- Demyelination – most common
- Sinus-related (ethmoiditis)
- Lyme disease

**Papillitis**

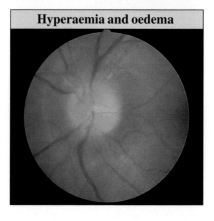

**Hyperaemia and oedema**

- Viral infections and immunization in children (bilateral)
- Demyelination (uncommon)
- Syphilis

**Neuroretinitis**

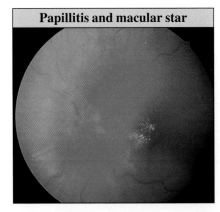

**Papillitis and macular star**

*Causes*
- **Cat-scratch fever**
- **Lyme disease**
- **Syphilis**

## 4. Anterior ischaemic optic neuropathy

**Non-arteritic**

| Presentation |
|---|
| ● **Age – 45–65 years** |
| ● **Altitudinal field defect** |
| ● **Eventually bilateral in 30% (give aspirin)** |

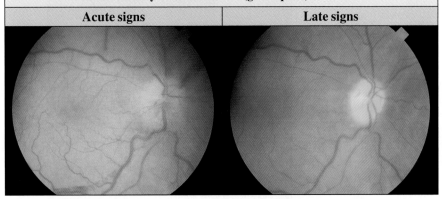

| Acute signs | Late signs |
|---|---|
| ● **Pale disc with diffuse or sectorial oedema**<br>● **Few, small splinter-shaped haemorrhages** | ● **Resolution of oedema and haemorrhages**<br>● **Optic atrophy and variable visual loss** |

## Fluorescence angiogram

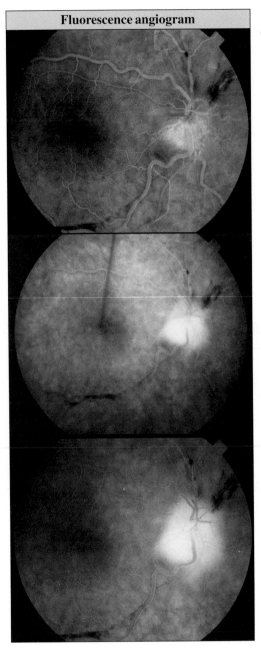

- Localized hyperfluorescence

- Increasing localized hyperfluorescence

- Generalized hyperfluorescence

**Arteritic**

- Affects about 25% of untreated patients with giant cell arteritis
- Severe acute visual loss
- Treatment – steroids to protect fellow eye
- Bilateral in 65% if untreated

## Signs

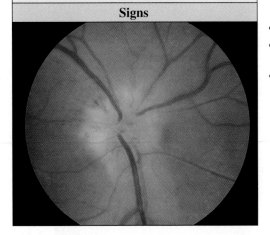

- Pale disc with diffuse oedema
- Few, small splinter-shaped haemorrhages
- Subsequent optic atrophy

## Superficial temporal arteritis

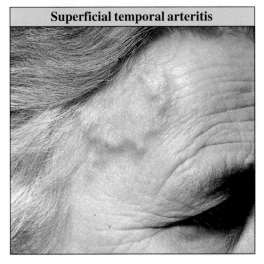

*Presentation*
- Age – 65–80 years
- Scalp tenderness
- Headache
- Jaw claudication
- Polymyalgia rheumatica
- Superficial temporal arteritis
- Acute visual loss

*Special investigations*
- ESR – often > 60, but normal in 20%
- C-reactive protein – always raised
- Temporal artery biopsy

## Histology of giant cell arteritis (1)

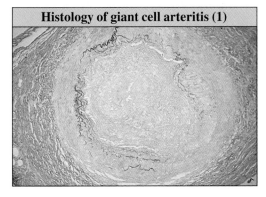

- Granulomatous cell infiltration
- Disruption of internal elastic lamina
- Proliferation of intima
- Occlusion of lumen

**Histology of giant cell arteritis (2)**

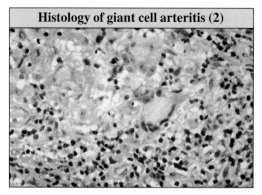

- High magnification shows giant cells

## 5. Leber hereditary optic neuropathy

- Maternal mitochondrial DNA mutations

**Signs**

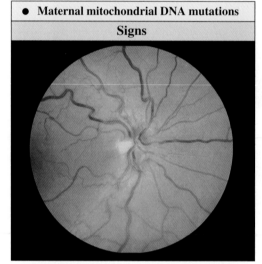

*Presentation*
- Typically in males – third decade
- Occasionally in females – any age
- Initially unilateral visual loss
- Fellow eye involved within 2 months
- Bilateral optic atrophy

- Disc hyperaemia and dilated capillaries (telangiectatic microangiopathy)
- Vascular tortuosity
- Swelling of peripapillary nerve fibre layer
- Subsequent bilateral optic atrophy

# PAPILLOEDEMA

## 1. Introduction
- Circulation of cerebrospinal fluid
- Causes of raised intracranial pressure
- Hydrocephalus

## 2. Classification of papilloedema
- Early
- Established (acute)
- Longstanding (chronic)
- Atrophic (secondary optic atrophy)

# 1. Introduction

### Circulation of cerebrospinal fluid

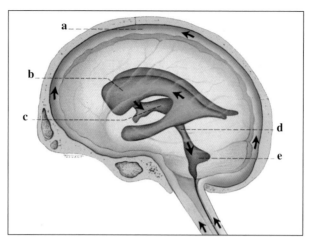

- Subarachnoid space (a)
- Lateral ventricle (b)
- Third ventricle (c)
- Aqueduct (d)
- Fourth ventricle (e)

### Causes of raised intracranial pressure

1. Space-occupying lesions
2. Blockage of ventricular system
3. Obstruction of CSF absorption
4. Benign intracranial hypertension (pseudotumour cerebri)
5. Diffuse cerebral oedema
6. Hypersecretion of CSF

### Hydrocephalus

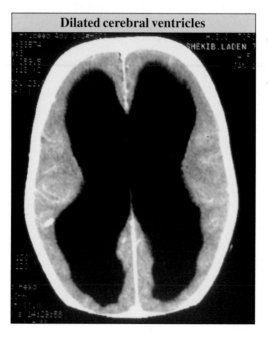

Dilated cerebral ventricles

- Communicating – obstruction to CSF flow in basilar cisterns or cerebral subarachnoid space
- Non-communicating – obstruction to CSF flow in ventricular system or at exit of foramina of fourth ventricle

## 2. Classification of papilloedema

**Early**

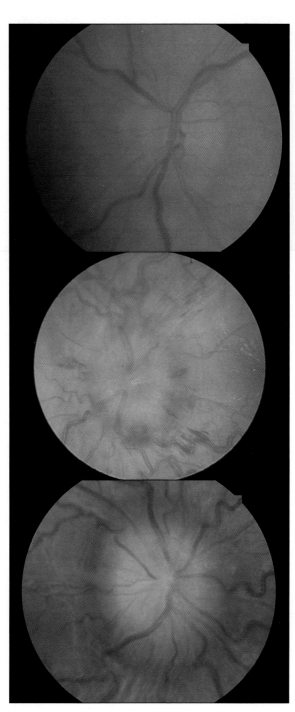

- VA – normal
- Mild disc hyperaemia
- Indistinct disc margins – initially nasal
- Mild venous engorgement
- Normal optic cup
- Spontaneous venous pulsation – absent (also absent in 20% of normals)

**Established (acute)**

- VA – usually normal
- Severe disc elevation and hyperaemia
- Very indistinct disc margins
- Obscuration of small vessels on disc
- Marked venous engorgement
- Reduced or absent optic cup
- Haemorrhages ± cotton-wool spots
- Macular star

**Longstanding (chronic)**

- VA – variable
- Marked disc elevation but less hyperaemia
- Disc margins – indistinct
- Variable venous engorgement
- Absent optic cup

**Atrophic (secondary optic atrophy)**

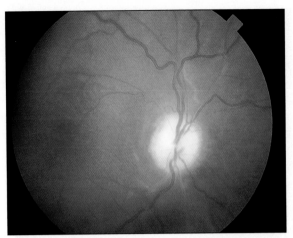

- VA – severely decreased
- Mild disc elevation
- Indistinct disc margins
- Disc pallor with few crossing vessels
- Absent optic cup

# CONGENITAL OPTIC NERVE ANOMALIES

1. **Without systemic associations**
   - Tilted optic disc
   - Optic disc drusen
   - Optic disc pit
   - Myelinated nerve fibres

2. **With systemic associations**
   - Optic disc coloboma
   - Morning glory anomaly
   - Optic nerve hypoplasia
   - Aicardi syndrome
   - Megalopapilla
   - Peripapillary staphyloma
   - Optic disc dysplasia

## 1. Without systemic associations

### Tilted optic disc

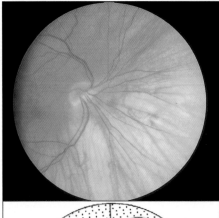

- VA – normal
- Common, bilateral
- Frequent myopia and astigmatism
- Small disc, oval or D-shaped
- Axis oblique (most common), horizontal or vertical
- Situs inversus and inferior crescent
- Hypopigmented inferonasal fundus

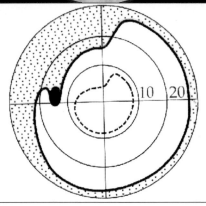

- Superotemporal field defects not obeying vertical midline

### Optic disc drusen

- Uncommon, bilateral and familial
- Associations – RP, angioid streaks and Alagille syndrome
- VA – usually normal

**Buried drusen**

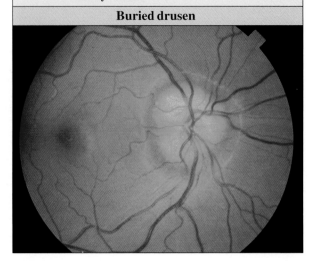

- Absent optic cup
- Pink or yellow colour
- Indistinct 'lumpy' margins
- Anomalous branching patterns with premature branching
- Absent venous engorgement

| Exposed | Occasional complications |
|---|---|

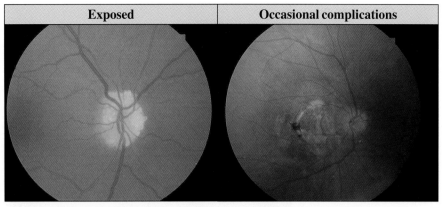

- Emergence from disc surface during early 'teens'
- Waxy pearl-like irregularities

- Choroidal neovascularization
- Nerve fibre bundle defects

## Fluorescein angiogram

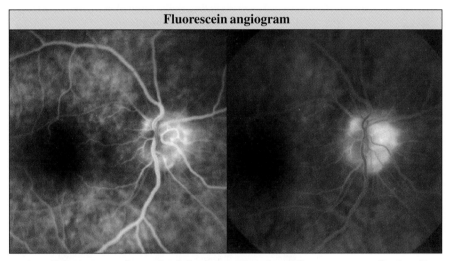

- Autofluorescence prior to dye injection
- Late hyperfluorescence confined to disc

| Imaging | |
|---|---|
| Ultrasonography | CT |

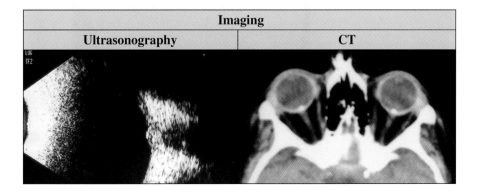

**Optic disc pit**

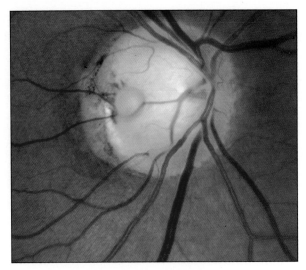

- Uncommon, usually unilateral
- VA – normal if uncomplicated
- Large disc containing round or oval pit
- Pit is usually temporal, occasionally central

| Macular detachment |
|---|
| • Incidence – 45% of non-central pits |
| • Initially – schisis-like separation of inner layers |
| • Later – serous detachment of outer layers |

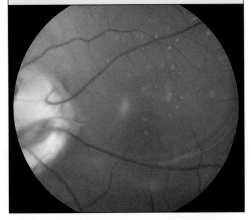

*Treatment*
- Laser photocoagulation to temporal disc
- Vitrectomy and gas tamponade if unresponsive

**Myelinated nerve fibres**

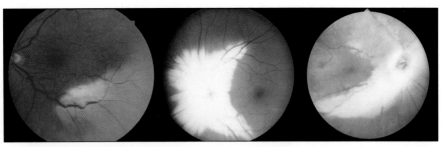

- Isolated peripheral
- Peripapillary
- Extensive

## 2. With systemic associations

**Optic disc coloboma**

- Rare, unilateral or bilateral
- Usually sporadic – occasionally dominant
- VA – decreased

| Signs | Ocular associations |
|---|---|

- Large disc with inferior excavation
- Superior visual field defects
- May be associated with other colobomas

### OCCASIONAL SYSTEMIC ASSOCIATIONS

1. CNS malformation – basal encephalocele and cysts
2. Chromosomal anomalies – Patau syndrome (trisomy 13) and cat-eye syndrome (trisomy 22)
3. 'CHARGE' – Coloboma, Heart defects, choanal Atresia, Retarded development, Genital and Ear anomalies
4. Other syndromes – Meckel–Gruber, Goltz, Lenz microphthalmos, Walker–Warburg and Goldenhar

**Morning glory anomaly**

- Very rare, usually unilateral
- VA – decreased

| Signs | Systemic association |
|---|---|

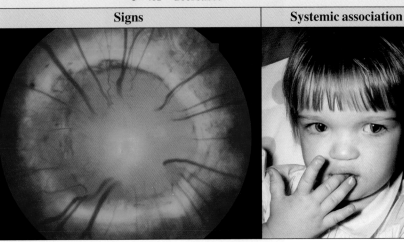

- Large disc with funnel-shaped excavation
- Glial tissue within base
- Spoke-like emerging vessels
- Surrounding chorioretinal pigmentary disturbance
- Serous retinal detachment in about 30%

- Basal encephalocele which is frequently associated with mid-facial anomalies

**Optic nerve hypoplasia**

- Rare, unilateral or bilateral
- VA – variable according to severity

| Signs | Systemic association |
|---|---|

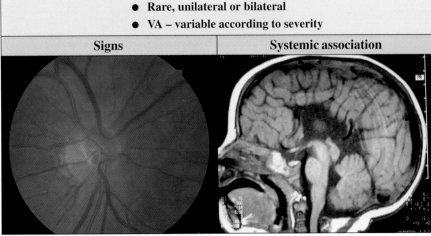

- Small disc surrounded by halo (double ring sign)
- Vessel normal calibre but may be tortuous

- De Morsier syndrome (septo-optic dysplasia)
- Absence of septum pellucidum and corpus callosum

**Aicardi syndrome**

- Very rare
- X-linked dominant which is lethal *in utero* for males
- Infantile spasms
- Developmental delay
- CNS malformations and early demise

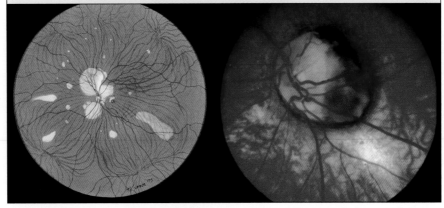

- Multiple 'chorioretinal lacunae'   •  Disc coloboma and pigmentation

**Megalopapilla**

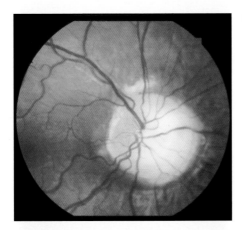

- Horizontal and vertical disc diameters over 2 mm

**Peripapillary staphyloma**

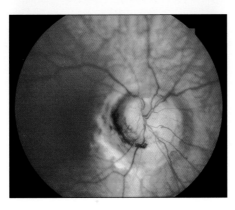

- Relatively normal disc within deep peripapillary excavation

**Optic disc dysplasia**

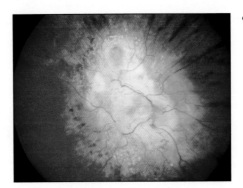

- Marked non-specific disc deformity

# OCULAR MOTOR NERVE PALSIES

1.  **Third nerve**

2.  **Fourth nerve**

3.  **Sixth nerve**

## 1. Third nerve

### Anatomy

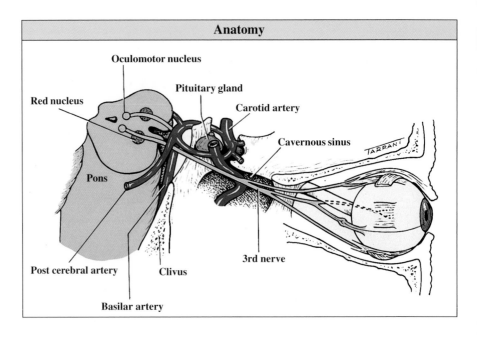

- Oculomotor nucleus
- Red nucleus
- Pituitary gland
- Carotid artery
- Cavernous sinus
- Pons
- 3rd nerve
- Post cerebral artery
- Clivus
- Basilar artery

### Applied anatomy of pupillomotor nerve fibres

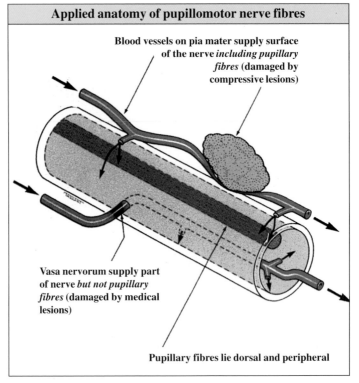

Blood vessels on pia mater supply surface of the nerve *including pupillary fibres* (damaged by compressive lesions)

Vasa nervorum supply part of nerve *but not pupillary fibres* (damaged by medical lesions)

Pupillary fibres lie dorsal and peripheral

## Sign of right third nerve palsy

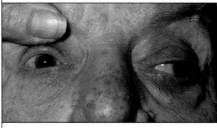

- Ptosis, mydriasis and cycloplegia
- Abduction in primary position

- Normal abduction
- Intorsion on attempted downgaze

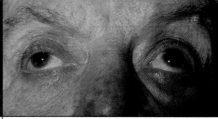

- Limited adduction

- Limited elevation

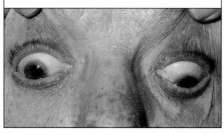

- Limited depression

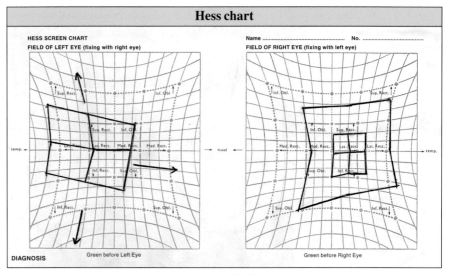

**Hess chart**

HESS SCREEN CHART
FIELD OF LEFT EYE (fixing with right eye)

FIELD OF RIGHT EYE (fixing with left eye)

Name ................................................ No. ..............

DIAGNOSIS — Green before Left Eye — Green before Right Eye

- Contraction of right chart and expansion of left
- Right chart – underactions of all muscles except lateral rectus and superior oblique
- Left chart – overactions of all muscles except medial rectus and inferior oblique

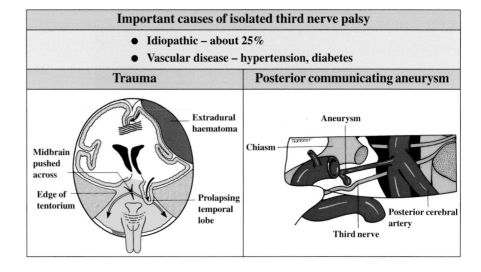

| Important causes of isolated third nerve palsy | |
|---|---|
| • Idiopathic – about 25% | |
| • Vascular disease – hypertension, diabetes | |
| **Trauma** | **Posterior communicating aneurysm** |

Extradural haematoma

Midbrain pushed across

Edge of tentorium

Prolapsing temporal lobe

Aneurysm

Chiasm

Posterior cerebral artery

Third nerve

## 2. Fourth nerve

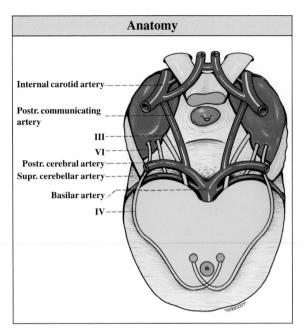

**Anatomy**

- Internal carotid artery
- Postr. communicating artery
- III
- VI
- Postr. cerebral artery
- Supr. cerebellar artery
- Basilar artery
- IV

- Only cranial nerve to emerge dorsally
- Crossed cranial nerve
- Very long and slender

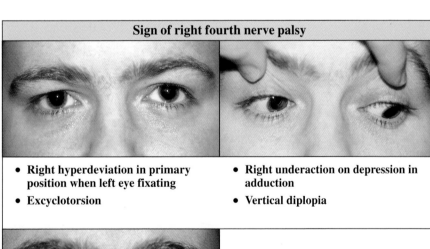

**Sign of right fourth nerve palsy**

- Right hyperdeviation in primary position when left eye fixating
- Excyclotorsion

- Right underaction on depression in adduction
- Vertical diplopia

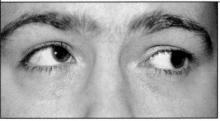

- Right overaction on left gaze

## Positive Bielschowsky test

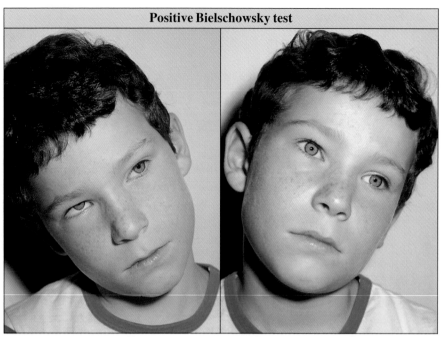

- Increase in right hyperdeviation on ipsilateral head tilt
- Absence of right hyperdeviation on contralateral head tilt

## Hess chart

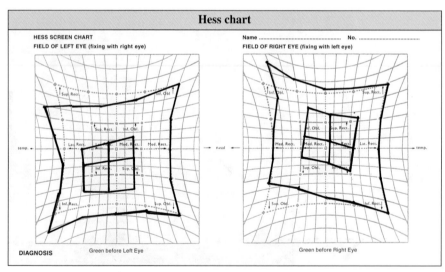

- No significant difference in chart size
- Upward deviation of right fixation spot on inner chart (hypertropia)
- Downward deviation of left fixation spot on inner chart
- Right chart – underaction of superior oblique and overaction of inferior oblique
- Left chart – overaction of inferior rectus and underaction of superior rectus

## 3. Sixth nerve

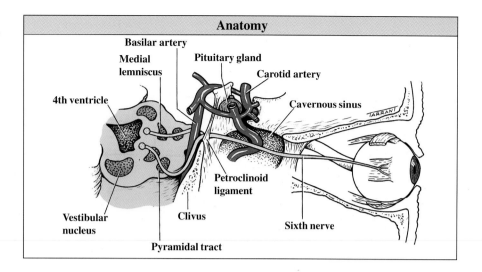

**Anatomy**

Basilar artery
Medial lemniscus
Pituitary gland
Carotid artery
4th ventricle
Cavernous sinus
Petroclinoid ligament
Vestibular nucleus
Clivus
Sixth nerve
Pyramidal tract

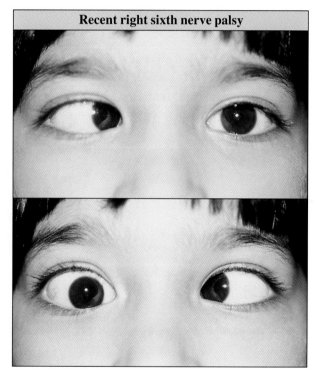

**Recent right sixth nerve palsy**

- Right esotropia in primary position due to unopposed action of right medial rectus

- Marked limitation of right abduction due to right lateral rectus weakness

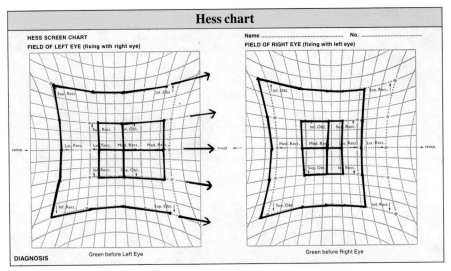

## Hess chart

**HESS SCREEN CHART**

FIELD OF LEFT EYE (fixing with right eye)

FIELD OF RIGHT EYE (fixing with left eye)

Name ............................................ No. ............................

temp. ←                    → nasal          nasal ←                    → temp.

Green before Left Eye

Green before Right Eye

DIAGNOSIS

- Contraction of right chart and expansion of left
- Right chart – marked underaction of lateral rectus and mild overaction of medial rectus
- Left chart – marked overaction of medial rectus

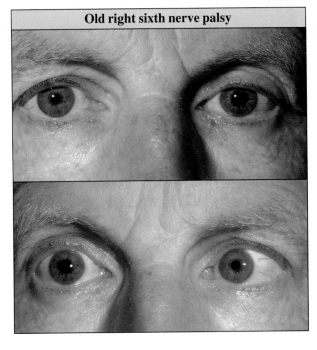

## Old right sixth nerve palsy

- Straight in primary position due to partial recovery

- Limitation of right abduction and horizontal diplopia

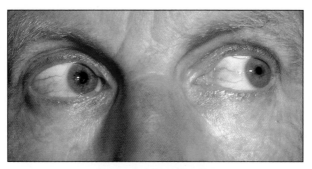

- Normal right adduction

| Important causes of isolated sixth nerve palsy |
|---|
| ● Vascular – hypertension, diabetes |

| Raised intracranial pressure | Acoustic neuroma |
|---|---|

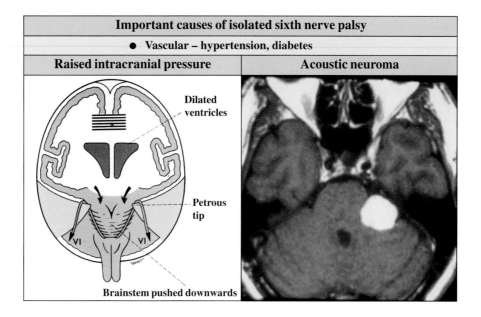

# DISORDERS OF THE CHIASM

1. **Anatomy**

2. **Pituitary adenomas**
   - Basophil adenoma
   - Acidophil adenoma
   - Chromophobe adenoma

3. **Craniopharyngioma**

4. **Meningioma**

## The chiasm and pituitary gland

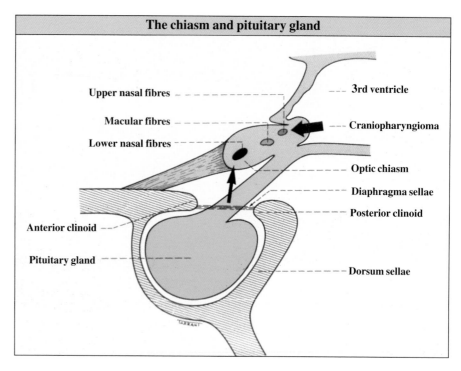

Upper nasal fibres — 3rd ventricle
Macular fibres — Craniopharyngioma
Lower nasal fibres — Optic chiasm
— Diaphragma sellae
— Posterior clinoid
Anterior clinoid —
Pituitary gland —
— Dorsum sellae

## Normal variations

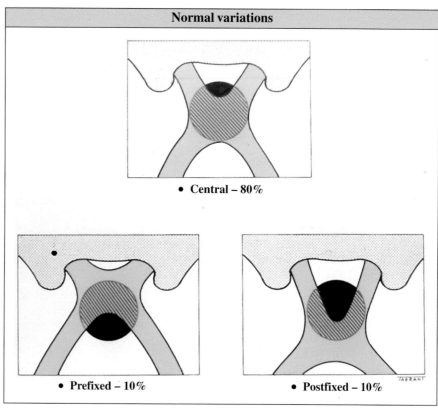

- Central – 80%
- Prefixed – 10%
- Postfixed – 10%

## 2. Pituitary adenomas

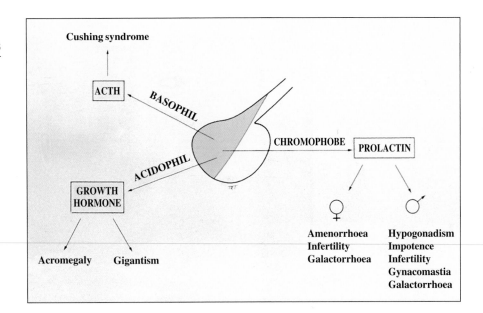

**Basophil adenoma**

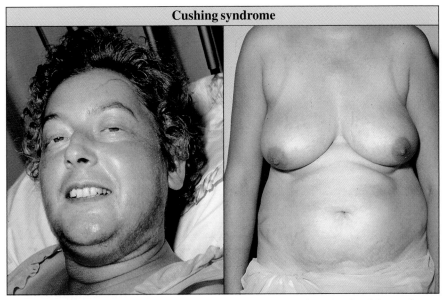

Cushing syndrome

- Moon face, pigmentation and hirsutism
- Hypertension and diabetes

- Obesity, skin striae, bruising and muscle weakness
- Ankle oedema and osteoporosis

**Acidophil adenoma**

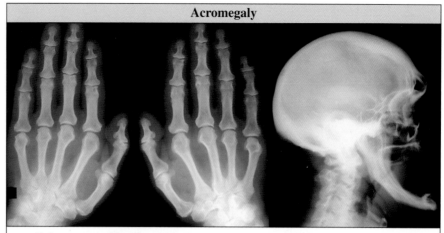

**Acromegaly**

- Enlargement of hands and feet
- Enlargement of lower jaw

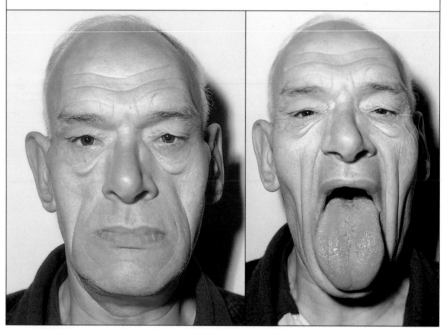

- Facial coarseness
- Hypertension, diabetes and gonadal dysfunction

- Organomegaly
- Carpal tunnel syndrome and cardiomyopathy

## Visual field defects

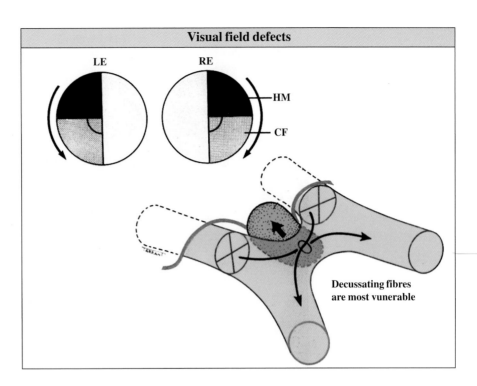

LE      RE

HM

CF

Decussating fibres
are most vunerable

## MRI scan (1)

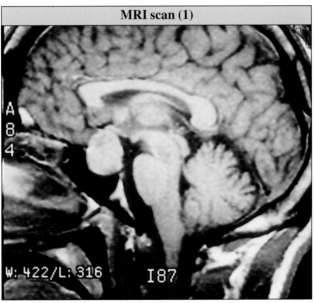

A
8
4

W:422/L:316   I87

- Sagittal

## MRI scan (2)

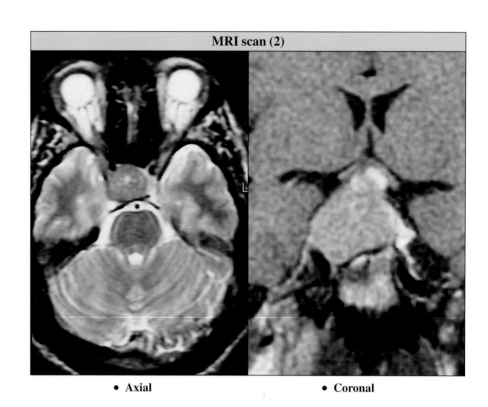

• Axial     • Coronal

## Treatment options

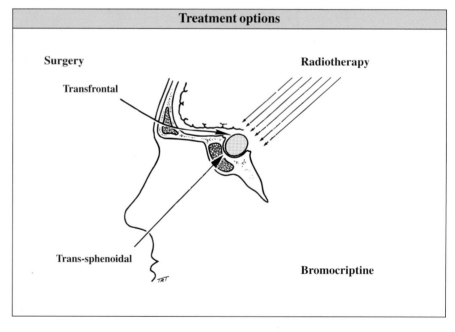

Surgery

Transfrontal

Trans-sphenoidal

Radiotherapy

Bromocriptine

## 3. Craniopharyngioma

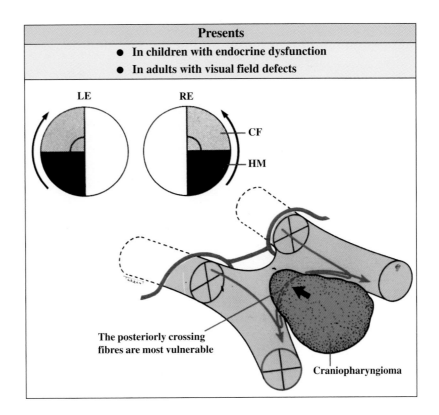

| Presents |
| --- |
| • In children with endocrine dysfunction |
| • In adults with visual field defects |

LE    RE

CF

HM

The posteriorly crossing
fibres are most vulnerable

Craniopharyngioma

## 4. Meningioma

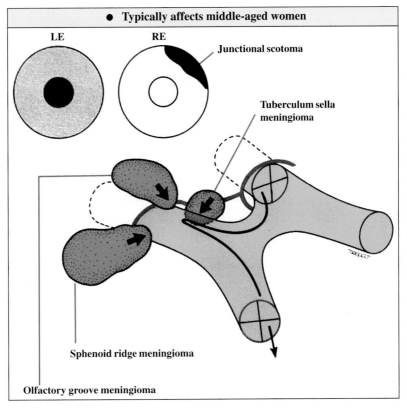

| • Typically affects middle-aged women |
| --- |

LE    RE

Junctional scotoma

Tuberculum sella
meningioma

Sphenoid ridge meningioma

Olfactory groove meningioma

# PHACOMATOSES

1. **Neurofibromatosis**
   - Type I (NF-1) – von Recklinghausen disease
   - Type II (NF-2) – bilateral acoustic neuromas

2. **Tuberous sclerosis (Bourneville disease)**

3. **von Hippel–Lindau syndrome**

4. **Sturge–Weber syndrome**

## 1. Neurofibromatosis

**Type I (NF-1)–von Recklinghausen disease**

- Most common phacomatosis
- Affects 1:4000 individuals
- Presents in childhood
- Gene localized to chromosome 17q11

### Café-au-lait spots

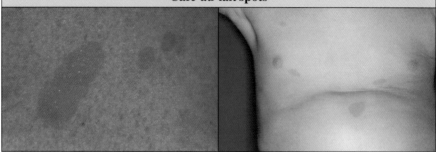

- Appear during first year of life
- Increase in size and number throughout childhood

### Fibroma molluscum

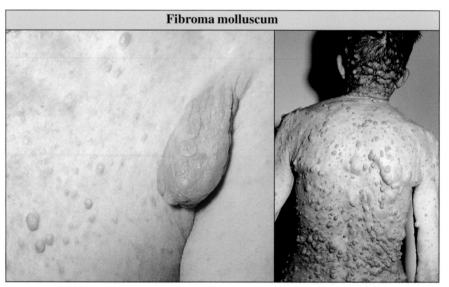

- Appear at puberty
- Pedunculated, flabby nodules consisting of neurofibromas or schwannomas
- Increase in number throughout life
- Frequently widely distributed

## Plexiform neurofibroma

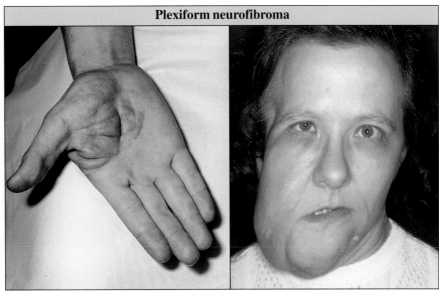

- Appear during childhood
- Large and ill-defined

- May be associated with overgrowth of overlying skin

## Skeletal defects

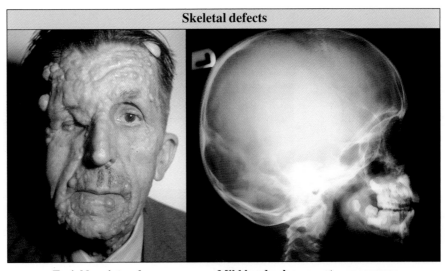

- Facial hemiatrophy

- Mild head enlargement – uncommon
- Other – scoliosis, short stature, thinning of long bones

| Orbital lesions | |
| --- | --- |
| Optic nerve glioma in about 15% | Spheno-orbital encephalocele |

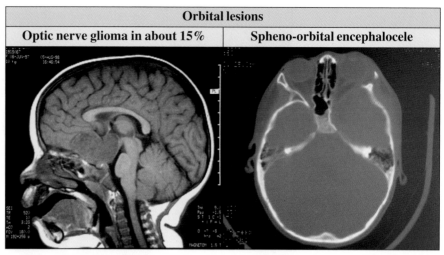

- Sagittal MRI scan of optic nerve glioma invading hypothalamus
- Glioma may be unilateral or bilateral

- Axial CT scan of congenital absence of left greater wing of sphenoid bone
- Causes pulsating proptosis without bruit

| Eyelid neurofibromas | |
| --- | --- |
| Nodular | Plexiform |

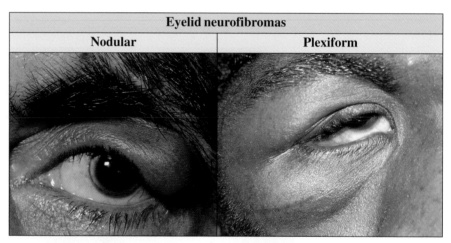

- May cause mechanical ptosis

- May be associated with glaucoma

| Intraocular lesions | |
|---|---|
| **Lisch nodules** | **Congenital ectropion uveae** |

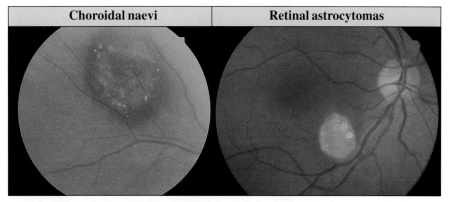

- Very common – eventually present in 95% of cases
- Uncommon – may be associated with glaucoma

| **Choroidal naevi** | **Retinal astrocytomas** |
|---|---|

- Common – may be multifocal and bilateral
- Rare – identical to those seen in tuberous sclerosis

**Type II (NF-2) – bilateral acoustic neuromas**

| Ocular features | |
|---|---|

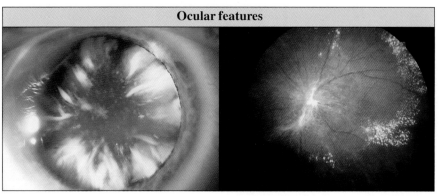

- Very common – presenile cataract
- Common – combined hamartomas of RPE and retina

## 2. Tuberous sclerosis (Bourneville disease)

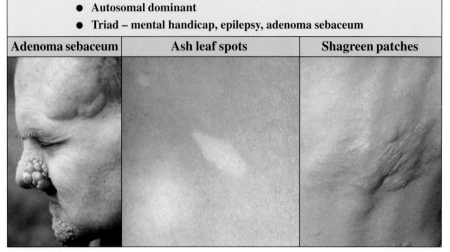

- Autosomal dominant
- Triad – mental handicap, epilepsy, adenoma sebaceum

| Adenoma sebaceum | Ash leaf spots | Shagreen patches |
|---|---|---|
| • Around nose and cheeks<br>• Appear after age 1 and slowly enlarge | • Hypopigmented skin patches<br>• In infants best detected using ultraviolet light (Wood's lamp) | • Diffuse thickening over lumbar region<br>• Present in 40% |

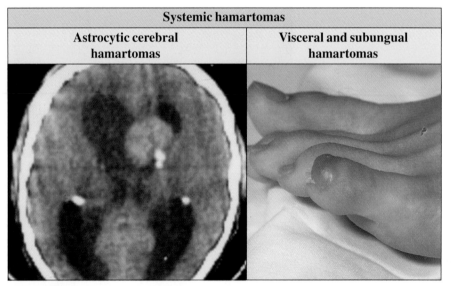

| Systemic hamartomas | |
|---|---|
| Astrocytic cerebral hamartomas | Visceral and subungual hamartomas |
| • Slow-growing periventricular tumours<br>• May cause hydrocephalus, epilepsy and mental retardation | • Usually asymptomatic and innocuous<br>• Kidneys (angiomyolipoma), heart (rhabdomyoma) |

| Retinal astrocytomas |
|---|
| ● Innocuous tumours present in 50% of patients<br>● May be multiple and bilateral |
| **Early** |

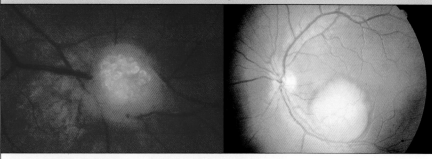

| ● Semitranslucent nodule | ● White plaque |
|---|---|

| **Advanced** |
|---|

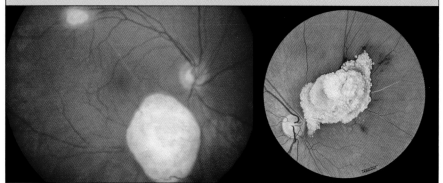

● Dense white tumour          ● Mulberry-like tumour

**3. von Hippel–Lindau syndrome**

| Systemic features |
|---|
| ● Autosomal dominant |

| CNS haemangioblastoma | Visceral tumours |
|---|---|
| 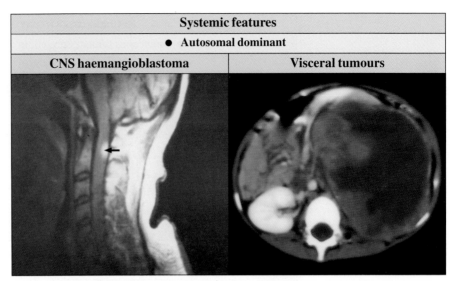 | |

● MRI of spinal cord tumour

● Tumours – renal carcinoma and phaeochromocytoma
● Cysts – kidneys, liver, pancreas, epididymis, ovary and lungs
● Polycythaemia

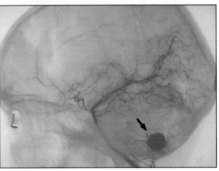

● Angiogram of cerebellar tumour

| Retinal capillary haemangioma |
|---|
| ● Vision-threatening tumour present in 50% of patients |
| ● May be multiple and bilateral |
| Early |

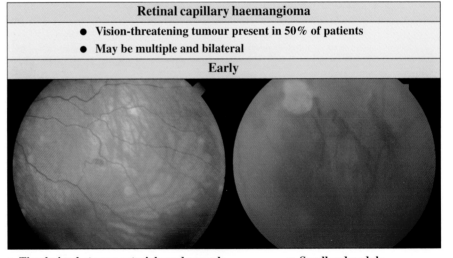

● Tiny lesion between arteriole and venuole          ● Small red nodule

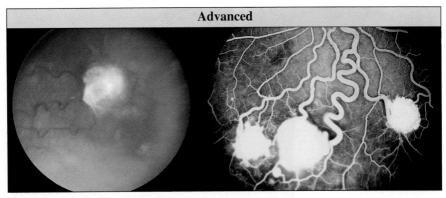

- Round orange-red mass
- Associated dilatation and tortuosity of feeder vessels

**Complications of retinal capillary haemangioma**

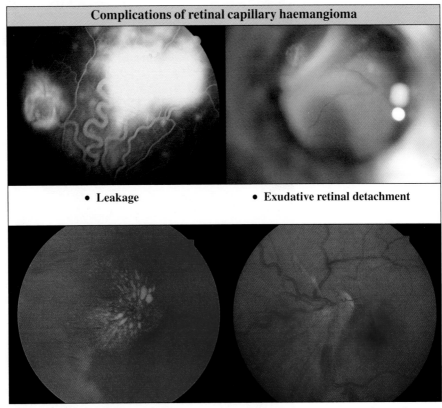

- Leakage
- Exudative retinal detachment

- Hard exudate formation
- Epiretinal membrane formation

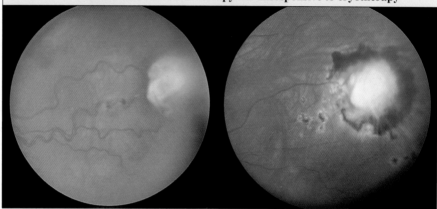

**Treatment options of retinal capillary haemangioma**

- Argon laser photocoagulation – small peripheral tumours
- Cryotherapy – larger peripheral tumours
- External beam radiotherapy – if unresponsive to cryotherapy

- Before treatment – dilated feeder vessels
- Following treatment – normal feeder vessels

## 4. Sturge–Weber syndrome

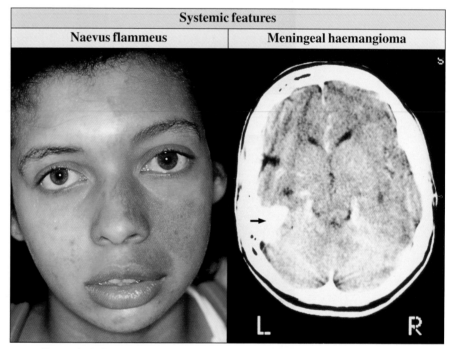

| Systemic features | |
|---|---|
| **Naevus flammeus** | **Meningeal haemangioma** |

- Congenital, does not blanch with pressure
- Associated with ipsilateral glaucoma in 30% of cases

- CT scan showing left parietal haemangioma
- Complications – mental handicap, epilepsy and hemiparesis

| Ocular features |
|---|
| **Glaucoma** |

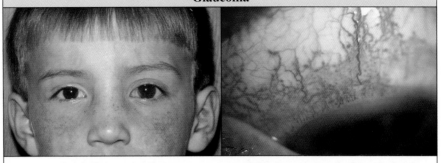

| • Buphthalmos in 60% | • May be associated with episcleral haemangioma |
|---|---|

| **Diffuse choroidal haemangioma** |
|---|

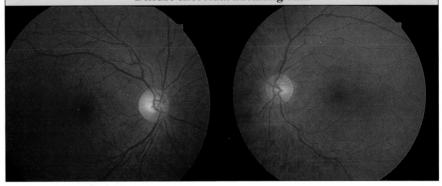

| • Normal eye | • Affected eye |
|---|---|

# Index